WORKBOOK TO ACCOMPANY

THE MEDICAL ASSISTANT

FIFTH EDITION

MARIAN G. COOPER, CMA-C

Past-President of the American Association of Medical Assistants;
Former Chairman of the American Association of Medical Assistants'
Curriculum Review Committee and Continuing Education Board.

DAVID E. COOPER, BS Ed.; ML

McGraw-Hill Book Company

New York   St. Louis   San Francisco   Auckland   Bogotá   Hamburg
London   Madrid   Mexico   Montreal   New Delhi
Panama   Paris   São Paulo   Singapore   Sydney   Tokyo   Toronto

NOTICE

As new medical and nursing research and clinical experience broaden our knowledge, changes in treatment and drug therapy are required. The editors and the publisher of this work have made every effort to ensure that the drug dosage schedules herein are accurate and in accord with the standards accepted at the time of publication. Readers are advised, however, to check the product information sheet included in the package of each drug they plan to administer to be certain that changes have not been made in the recommended dose or in the contraindications for administration. This recommendation is of particular importance in regard to new or infrequently used drugs.

Workbook to Accompany
THE MEDICAL ASSISTANT
Fifth Edition

Copyright © 1970, 1978, 1986 by McGraw-Hill, Inc. All rights reserved. Printed in the United States of America. No part of this publication may be reproduced, stored in a retrieval system, or transmitted, in any form or by any means electronic, mechanical, photocopying, recording, or otherwise, without the prior written permission of the publisher.

ISBN 0-07-012757-3

67890 SEMSEM

The editor was Sally J. Barhydt;
the production supervisor was Charles Hess;
the cover was designed by Rafael Hernandez.
Semline, Inc., was printer and binder.

CONTENTS

TO THE STUDENT

This workbook has been prepared for those of you who use *The Medical Assistant* s a textbook. The sections of the workbook are numbered and titled to match the hapters of the text.

The questions and work projects which follow will serve to test your knowledge. n addition, they are designed to stimulate thought and thus help you to develop a reater familiarity with and a deeper understanding of the subject. In some spots he material goes beyond the information contained in the text in order to encourage ou to use additional references and to think for yourself. Use of the workbook in onjunction with the text should facilitate and enhance the overall learning process.

Marian G. Cooper

David E. Cooper

CHAPTER 1

MEDICAL ASSISTING—THE OCCUPATION

UIZ

. Answer each of the following questions in the space provided:

1. Briefly state the basic purpose of the medical assisting occupation.

   _____

   _____

2. What are the two general categories of duties performed by medical assistants?

   _____

   _____

3. Name five job specialties that are encompassed in the broad definition of medical assistant.

   1. _____

   2. _____

   3. _____

   4. _____

   5. _____

   _____

   _____

   _____

4. The AAMA works jointly with the _____

   _____ in the accreditation of medical assisting

   educational programs.

5. About how many medical assistants are there in the United States?

   _____

6. Name at least seven duties of a business nature that a medical assistant might be expected to perform:

   1. _____

   2. _____

   3. _____

   4. _____

   5. _____

   6. _____

   7. _____

   8. _____

   9. _____

   10. _____

   11. _____

   12. _____

7. Name at least five duties of a medical nature that a medical assistant might be expected to perform:

   1. _____

   2. _____

   3. _____

   4. _____

   5. _____

   6. _____

   7. _____

   8. _____

   9. _____

8. Name two national professional organizations for medical assistants.

_____

_____

9. Each of the above professional organizations has a credentialing program to recognize competence in the medical assisting field. Those passing the required examination are known as:

_____

_____

PRACTICE AND PROJECTS

Make a list of those duties of a medical assistant that are most appealing to you.

_____

_____

_____

_____

_____

_____

Write your opinion of the future of medical assisting. (Maximum 100 words.)

_____

_____

_____

_____

_____

_____

_____

_____

C. Why do you think it is important to become certified or registered as a medical assistant? (Maximum 100 words.)

_____

_____

_____

_____

_____

_____

_____

MEDICAL ASSISTANT—
THE INDIVIDUAL

This section is not a test of text material but for your personal self-analysis.
ou may be asked to answer these questions as you begin your medical assisting train-
ng and again as you complete it. You should be completely honest in your answers
s they are for your benefit for a better understanding of yourself.

There are no passing or failing scores.

JIZ

n each of the following questions check the answer that is most correct for you.

. How long have you had an interest in working in the field of medicine?

1. _____ Many years

2. _____ Several years

3. _____ Several months

4. _____ As yet uncertain

. How important is it to you that your job involve helping other people?

1. _____ Would not accept any other kind of job.

2. _____ Would prefer a job that involves directly helping others but would
accept other appealing work.

3. _____ Would accept any type of work with good salary and working conditions.

. In your day-to-day work would you prefer to:

1. _____ be in frequent direct contact with patients?

2. _____ have some direct contact with patients?

3. _____ work primarily with other office personnel?

4. _____ work mostly in privacy?

D. If you were dealing with a patient who was overly demanding and critical, would you try to:

1. _____ maintain your composure and treat the patient as much as possible as you would any other patient?

2. _____ do what is necessary for the patient but with as little contact as possible?

3. _____ treat the patient as he or she treats you?

E. After you have begun to work as a medical assistant, would you:

1. _____ take additional courses and/or participate in workshops to keep up-to date and learn about new developments?

2. _____ be content to keep abreast of new developments by scanning professional magazines and talking with fellow medical assistants?

3. _____ assume that additional study is unnecessary if your employer seems satisfied with your work?

F. What most nearly describes your feelings at the present time regarding how you would like to be able to conduct yourself if confronted with an emergency situation in which someone was injured?

1. _____ Would want to be familiar with basic emergency procedures in order to be as much immediate help as possible.

2. _____ Would call the closest hospital or medical-emergency service.

3. _____ Would avoid participation in emergency care in view of limited knowledge of correct action to take.

G. When given a job assignment in which accuracy is important, would you:

1. _____ discipline yourself to do all phases of the job as perfectly as you know how?

2. _____ be concerned about the critical phases of the work and save time on the others?

3. _____ concentrate on those features of the work that your supervisor would be able to review?

H. How would you characterize yourself regarding the following?

1. _____ Very particular about neatness and cleanliness at all times.

2. _____ Occasionally willing to take shortcuts in matters of cleanliness in order to save time.

3. _____ Particular in those aspects of cleanliness that are visible to others.

I. If your planned schedule of work as a medical assistant were interrupted several times in a morning due to emergencies, would you:

1. _____ recognize that this is expectable in a doctor's office and handle the more important matters first without becoming annoyed?

2. _____ handle the cases without trying to disguise your frustration?

6

3. _____ adhere to the schedule until the doctor directs otherwise?

If the doctor is interrupted while examining a patient, would you:

1. _____ explain the situation to the patient and make sure he or she is as comfortable as possible while waiting for the doctor to return?

2. _____ tell the patient that emergencies are to be expected and the doctor will return shortly?

3. _____ attend to other duties since the examination cannot proceed until the doctor returns?

nalysis results:

Write in the number of times you chose number 1, 2, 3, or 4.

1. _____   2. _____   3. _____   4. _____

If most of the answers are number 1, this would indicate a personality and set of values that are desirable in medical assistants.

RACTICE AND PROJECTS

. State briefly what led you to take this program in Medical Assisting.

_____

_____

_____

_____

. Make a list of at least ten (10) of your basic character traits and viewpoints that you feel will help you to be a first-class medical assistant.

1. _____

2. _____

3. _____

4. _____

5. _____

6. _____

7. _____

8. _____

9. _____

10. _____

CHAPTER 3

PROFESSIONAL STANDARDS— RELATIONSHIPS AND APPEARANCES

QUIZ

A. From the items listed under each question, select the correct answer or answers. Write the corresponding letter or letters in the answer space.

1. All of the following are important in dealing with patients except:

   a. treat each patient with full respect.
   b. consider the patient's desire for privacy.
   c. develop a standard way of handling all patients.
   d. consider each patient as an individual personality.

2. Which of the following is appropriate for the medical assistant in working relations with the doctor?

   a. Study the doctor's practices and preferences in order to anticipate his or her needs.
   b. Use the title "Doctor" with his or her name when referring to the doctor.
   c. Avoid any criticism of the doctor when talking with patients.
   d. Become proficient in your job so that you and the doctor can work together as a team.

3. A personnel review session is an appropriate time to discuss:

   a. purchasing a new piece of equipment.
   b. how well the medical assistant is performing his or her duties.
   c. how well the cleaning people are doing their work.
   d. the vacation schedule. _____

4. A good way to get along with fellow employees is to:

   a. avoid those you do not care for.
   b. report directly to the doctor any difficulties you may have with a fellow worker.
   c. be cooperative and talk and act in a way that brings out the best in others.
   d. do your own work and pay no attention to others. _____

5. If the doctor's spouse makes a suggestion about changing an office procedure, the best way to handle it would be to:

   a. say courteously that you cannot change the procedure unless the doctor tells you to.
   b. explain that you are doing it properly as you were taught.
   c. express appreciation for the suggestion and then discuss it with the doctor.
   d. explain that you are doing the procedure as the doctor instructed.

6. Proper personal appearance can be considered a requirement for a medical assistant for all of the following reasons except:

   a. medical work involves close contact with patients.
   b. patients will feel more confident about the medical care they receive.
   c. patients will expect to see office personnel who are aware of the latest style.
   d. patients will respond more readily to advice about their own care.

7. The main thing for a medical assistant to consider in a hair style is that it:

   a. is a currently popular style.
   b. will not require frequent adjustment during the working day.
   c. is a flattering length.
   d. is worn off the face.

8. To minimize the risk of transferring of infections, medical assistants should:

   a. wash their hands before and after handling a patient.
   b. wear nail polish to protect the nails.
   c. cover breaks or cuts in the skin before handling patients.
   d. use hand lotions frequently.

9. All of the following are important things to consider from a functional standpoint when selecting a uniform except:

   a. it is high fashion.
   b. the sleeves are close fitting.
   c. the material can be easily spot-cleaned.
   d. it allows for good freedom of movement.

10. The medical assistant's shoes should:

    a. be cleaned at the beginning of each day.
    b. have heels and soles that minimize noise.
    c. be comfortable according to the assistant's choice.
    d. be stylish.

1. List six medical assistant functions which involve direct contact with patients.

1. _____

2. _____

3. _____

4. _____

5. _____

6. _____

2. List four working conditions, aside from salary, starting and quitting times, which should be clearly understood at the beginning of employment.

1. _____ 3. _____

2. _____ 4. _____

3. Name eight types of people the medical assistant should be prepared to deal with other than patients, the doctor and his family, or other employees.

1. _____

2. _____

3. _____

4. _____

5. _____

6. _____

7. _____

8. _____

4. List four types of public service which medical assistants might volunteer to do.

1. _____

2. _____

3. _____

4. _____

5. What items of jewelry are always acceptable for a medical assistant to wear at work?

1. _____

2. _____

3. _____

PRACTICE AND PROJECTS

A. In one sentence state what you believe is the primary objective of medical personnel, including medical assistants.

_____

_____

B. List the things you feel you could do to enhance the medical assistant's image with the public.

_____

_____

_____

_____

_____

CHAPTER 4

MEDICAL LAW AND ETHICS

Complete the following sentences or answer the questions, using the blank spaces provided.

1. What are the statutes commonly called that deal with the licensing of physicians?

   Medical practice acts

2. Are the statutes dealing with licensing of physicians local, federal, or state laws?

   State

3. What is the nature of the legal relationship between a patient and a doctor?

   Contract

4. If a doctor moves to another state, must he or she obtain a license to practice in that state?

   Yes

5. What two conditions create a physician-patient contract?

   1. *offer*

   2. *acceptance*

6. When speaking or acting on behalf of the doctor, the medical assistant is legally acting as the doctor's _*agent*_ .

7. In a medical contract, what is the principal obligation of the patient?

   Provide doctor with complete + accurate info. *pay for services received*

8. In a physician-patient contract, does the patient's presentation of himself or herself for examination constitute his or her part of the contract agreement?

   Yes

13

9. When the doctor is called by a relative of a patient who is too ill to call, generally who is obligated to pay the fee?

Patient

10. Most physician-patient contracts are not written but instead are

implied.

11. The information that the doctor learns about a patient during examination and treatment is generally regarded as _Confidential_ and should not be passed on to others unless the patient _Consents_.

12. The law requires standards of performance for doctors. The medical profession has set for itself additional rules of conduct known as the

Principles of medical ethics.

B. From the items listed under each question, select the correct answer or answers. Write the corresponding letter or letters in the answer space.

1. Which of the following statements are correct in regard to renewal of a license to practice medicine?

   a. Renewal is not necessary as long as the physician remains in active practice.
   b. Periodic renewal is required.
   c. Proof of participation in continuing medical education is sometimes required.
   d. Fees are usually charged for renewal of a license to practice medicine.

   _B-C-D_

2. Which of the following would be grounds for revocation of a license?

   a. Excessive fees
   b. Refusal to treat a patient
   c. Refusal to care for Medicare patients
   d. Drug addiction

   _D_

3. Which of the following are correct in regard to a patient's consent to examination or treatment?

   a. Presenting oneself to a doctor and asking for care is sufficient indication of patient's consent to undergo routine and nonhazardous procedures.
   b. Written consent is not important if surgery is performed in the office.
   c. The patient must have been given a full and understandable explanation of the risks involved in order to have a signed consent form be legally valid.
   d. "Informed consent" means the patient consents only on the basis of full explanation and understanding of a medical

procedure and that there were no assurances of improved
health beyond those reasonably expectable.

    e. The patient's signature on a consent form is sufficient
to make the consent legally valid.   *A-C-D*

4. If a physician decides he no longer wishes to treat a patient,
which of the following is the proper procedure?

    a. Notify the patient in writing.
    b. Try to persuade the patient to see another doctor.
    c. Notify the patient, giving sufficient time to obtain
another physician, and advise if continued treatment
is necessary.   *C*

5. If a patient asks the medical assistant for his or her x-rays,
which of the following is the correct procedure?

    a. Give the x-rays to the patient.
    b. Ask for a signed release before giving the x-rays to the
patient.
    c. Advise the patient that the x-rays are the property of the
doctor, but offer to send them to another physician.
    d. Advise the patient that the x-rays are the property of the
doctor and cannot be released to anyone.   *B-C*

6. Which of the following require the consent of another person
before the doctor may begin treatment?

    a. Married woman
    b. Unconscious person requiring immediate treatment
    c. Married minor
    d. Incompetent person with a legal guardian
    e. Patient who refuses proper treatment   *D*

7. During an examination of a woman patient, a male doctor should
have a female medical assistant present. Which of the following
is the legal reason for this?

    a. To avoid later claims of malpractice
    b. To avoid later claims that the examination was conducted
without the patient's consent or that the doctor otherwise
acted improperly
    c. To reassure the patient and properly assist the doctor
    d. To assure proper protection of the patient's rights   *B-*

8. Malpractice refers to which of the following?

    a. Any instance where a doctor causes injury to a patient
    b. Failure of the doctor to apply the most advanced treatment
    c. Failure of the doctor to explain the prospects for
recovery to the patient
    d. Failure of the doctor through negligence to carry out his
or her legal duties to the patient and injury results   *D*

9. Which of the following should the medical assistant do if a patient asks for the results of tests?

    a. Inform the patient about those tests where the results are clear.
    b. Advise the patient that only the doctor can discuss test results.
    c. Ask the doctor if the results may be given out and, if so, make it clear to the patient that the information comes from the doctor.
    d. Tell the patient that the assistant is not permitted to give out test information.

    C

10. Rules of conduct that deal with the relationships between doctors come under the heading of which of the following?

    a. Medical etiquette
    b. Medical ethics
    c. Professional relations
    d. Public relations

    A

11. In which of the following can the medical assistant help the doctor meet the obligation of being reasonably available to patients?

    a. Know the daily schedule and how to reach the doctor in case of emergency.
    b. When the doctor is ill or out of town, know how to reach the other doctors who have agreed to handle the patients.
    c. Avoid overscheduling that may lead to the doctor's being unable to treat critical cases on time.
    d. All of the above.

    D

12. If a patient expresses dissatisfaction with the doctor's fee to the medical assistant, which of the following should the assistant do?

    a. Inform the doctor of the patient's dissatisfaction.
    b. Inform the patient that this is the doctor's usual fee.
    c. Tell the patient that you will ask the doctor about adjusting the fee.
    d. Inform the patient that the fee was set by the doctor and that the bill is correct.

    A

13. The doctor has a legal obligation to provide patients with a certain standard of care. Which of the following are descriptive of this standard?

    a. The doctor must have knowledge and skills at least equal to those of the average physician in similar types of practice.
    b. The doctor must use reasonable care in applying his or her skill and knowledge.
    c. The doctor must use his or her best judgment in treating each case.
    d. The patient must have some improvement in health.
    e. The patient must be satisfied with the care received.

    A-B C

1. Name three general educational or training requirements for persons seeking a license to practice medicine.

1. _Undergraduate Degree_
2. _① 4 years medical school — ② Internship Accredited Hosp._
3. _Certification on Medical Boards_

2. The medical assistant may properly handle and carry narcotic drugs under what condition.

Under Doctor's supervision & orders.

3. List at least five items that generally are covered in a medical practice act.

1. _Create State Board to administer for license_
2. _Define medical practice_
3. _List qualification for license — (educational & personal)_
4. _Outline steps for obtaining license_
5. _Identify improper behavior for revoking license_
6.

4. List three types of behavior on the part of a physician that may become the basis for a malpractice suit.

Inadequate diagnosis
1. _Drug and/or alcohol abuse_
Omission of standard treatment
2. _Failure to use ordinary care_
failure to refer patient to appropriate
3. _Unavailable when needed — Specialist_
Exposure to infection

5. Describe two situations in which a patient's freedom of movement may be legally restricted, and indicate the nature of the restraint.

SITUATION	FORM OF RESTRAINT
1. _Contagious disease_	_Quarantine_
2. _Mental disease_	_Mental Institution_

6. List three ways in which the medical assistant can help the doctor avoid malpractice suits.

1. _Keeping records completely, accurately, neatly_
Sterilization & maintaining equipment
2. _relay physicians instructions accurately_
& completely

17

3. _Don't treat, diagnose (overstep authority)_

7. List two types of tort liability to which the doctor could be subjected if information about the patient were improperly given out. Briefly define each type of tort.

TYPE OF TORT	DEFINITION
1. _Assault & Battery_	(1) _Testing or treating without consent. Doctor mistreatment_
(2) _Invasion of privacy_	(2) _Exposure of patient's person or records_
3. _Defamation –_	(3) _False statement – cause ridicule or damaged reputation_

8. List five types of occurrences that doctors are required by law to report to government authorities.

1. _Birth_   _Drug control_
2. _Death_   _Food poisoning_
3. _Injuries from child abuse or violence_   _Occupational injuries_
4. _Gunshot wounds_
5. _Infectious diseases_

9. List at least four requirements important from a legal point of view in preparing and maintaining medical records.

1. _Confidential – Complete_
2. _Accurate – legible_
3. _Written Consent for surgical procedures or releasing info._
4. _Promptness – well organized_

18

10. If a patient with a serious illness fails to keep an appointment, what should the doctor do from the legal viewpoint?

Write letter stating how important treatment - copy in file - try to schedule another appointment -

11. To stay clear of antitrust charges, physicians should not make agreements with other physicians with respect to certain aspects of medical practice. Three types of agreements which should be avoided are:

1. *Fix pricing*

2. *Allocate territories*

3. *Boycott*

12. Give the definition of implied consent.

Consent expressed in action or verbally but not expressly written -

PRACTICE AND PROJECTS

A. In the answer space below, compose a form for consent to a diagnostic procedure.

_____

_____

_____

_____

_____

_____

_____

B. Describe a situation that could result in a malpractice suit against the doctor because of negligence on the part of the medical assistant.

_____

_____

_____

_____

HANDLING MEDICAL
EMERGENCIES—FIRST AID

QUIZ

A. Complete the following sentences or answer the questions in the space provided.

1. An acknowledged authority on first aid is _____.

2. Medical assistants are expected to know more about first aid than the

   _____.

3. Does first aid include self-help in emergency situations? _____

4. In emergency situations requiring prompt attention, should the medical
   assistant undertake a tentative diagnosis when the doctor is not available?

   _____

5. In emergency situations requiring prompt attention, should the medical
   assistant proceed with first aid treatment when a doctor is not available?

   _____

6. When the doctor is present during a medical emergency, should the medical

   assistant attempt diagnosis and/or treatment? _____

7. Is sudden illness regarded as a medical emergency? _____

8. A tourniquet, once applied, should not be removed until the victim is in a

   location where he or she can be treated for _____.

9. In carbonmonoxide poisoning, the skin and lips are _____
   in color.

10. Cold water is the first aid treatment for _____ and _____
    degree burns.

11. When breathing has stopped, death can occur in _____ to _____ minutes.

12. Cardiopulmonary resuscitation, which is identified by the abbreviation
    _____, is a combination of artificial _____ and manual
    artificial _____.

21

13. One sign of imminent childbirth is contractions at _____ minute interval

B. From the items listed under each question or statement, select the correct answer or answers. Write the corresponding letter or letters in the answer space.

1. The general guidelines of a standard of behavior that a medical assistant should follow in a medical emergency situation are:

   a. give the kind of aid that others with similar training and experience might be expected to give.
   b. provide the type of aid referred to in (a) above with reasonable care.
   c. do not make a diagnosis or proceed with treatment.
   d. recognize the limits of your knowledge and do nothing that might cause further injury.

2. The general benefits that can be realized through the proper application of first aid include:

   a. a better chance for earlier recovery.
   b. lower immediate medical expenses.
   c. a lesser degree of ultimate disability.
   d. the saving of lives.

3. For light bleeding, what would be the proper first-aid measure?

   a. Elevate injured part as much as possible above heart level.
   b. Apply a tourniquet if bleeding continues.
   c. Draw flesh together and apply pressure with dressing directly over wound.
   d. Control bleeding by using pressure points.

4. If bleeding is so profuse that the dressing becomes soaked:

   a. use a new dry dressing.
   b. increase the pressure over the wound.
   c. add additional layers of dressing and continue direct pressure.
   d. use a pressure point distal to the wound.

5. In the first-aid treatment of a second-degree burn:

   a. blisters should be opened.
   b. the injured part should be submersed in cold water.
   c. dead tissue should be carefully removed.
   d. the burned area should be covered with an ointment.

6. For a chemical burn of the face and eyes, what first-aid procedure should be done first?

   a. Use anesthetic spray to relieve pain.
   b. Immerse in water as much as possible.
   c. Flood with continuous flow of water.
   d. Cover with dry dressing and have patient taken immediately to a hospital emergency unit.

22

7. What general first aid procedure is recommended in the case of a broken arm or leg?

    a. Attempt to straighten the injured part.
    b. Immobilize the injured part.
    c. Elevate the injured limb.
    d. Do not touch the affected limb and have the patient taken to the hospital as quickly as possible. _____

8. Insect stings can cause anaphylaxis. This would be of particular concern in certain individuals, such as:

    a. pregnant women.
    b. asthma patients.
    c. those who have had allergic reaction to bee stings.
    d. those with a history of allergies. _____

9. Symptoms of a stroke include:

    a. sudden collapse.
    b. partial paralysis.
    c. slurred speech.
    d. abdominal pain.
    e. pupils unequal in size. _____

10. Bandages may be used for the following first aid purposes:

    a. to apply pressure to control bleeding.
    b. to limit blood circulation.
    c. to immobilize an injured limb.
    d. to protect an injured area.
    e. to keep out dirt or other contaminants. _____

11. In the case of dog bite:

    a. tell the victim to wash the bite with soap and water.
    b. have victim massage the site.
    c. tell the victim to make every effort to identify the dog and see that it is confined until it can be determined if it is rabid.
    d. tell the victim to minimize movement of the affected part. _____

12. Which of the following represent normal childbirth?

    a. The back of the baby's head is usually the first part to be seen.
    b. The baby's face is usually down as birth begins.
    c. The baby's head turns to the side as it emerges.
    d. Support of the baby's head is necessary as the shoulders begin to emerge.
    e. Once the shoulders are through the birth canal, the remainder of the baby's body will come out quickly. _____

C. 1. List three basic steps of advance preparation that would be taken in most doctors' offices to be ready for medical emergencies.

1. _____

_____

2. _____

_____

3. _____

_____

2. For what emergency services would you have telephone numbers posted on or near your telephones? Name eight and look up and list the local numbers your community.

EMERGENCY SERVICE   **TELEPHONE NUMBE**

1. _____   1. _____

2. _____   2. _____

3. _____   3. _____

4. _____   4. _____

5. _____   5. _____

6. _____   6. _____

7. _____   7. _____

8. _____   8. _____

_____   _____

3. List six medical items that you would include in an office first aid kit.

1. _____

2. _____

3. _____

4. _____

5. _____

6. _____

_____

_____

4. Name and briefly describe the five kinds of wounds that cause external bleeding.

KIND OF WOUND	DESCRIPTION
1. _____	1. _____
2. _____	2. _____
3. _____	3. _____
4. _____	4. _____
5. _____	5. _____

5. Give two general rules for stopping or lessening external bleeding.

1. _____

2. _____

6. Name the artery and describe the location of the two most effective pressure points in the body.

ARTERY	LOCATION
1. _____	1. _____
	_____
	_____
2. _____	2. _____
	_____

7. List the three degrees of burns and briefly describe each.

BURN	DESCRIPTION
1. _____	1. _____
2. _____	2. _____
	_____
3. _____	3. _____
	_____

8. List four common symptoms of a heart attack.

1. _____

2. _____

3. _____

4. _____

9. List three common symptoms of shock resulting from injury:

1. _____

2. _____

3. _____

_____

PRACTICE AND PROJECTS

A. State in your own words a definition of first aid comparable to that given by The American National Red Cross.

_____

_____

_____

_____

_____

B. There are some general rules for administering first aid shown under the head of "FIRST AID PROCEDURES" in the text. Study these carefully and restate the in your own words and in the order in which they would generally apply in the average emergency situation. Add any general rules that you feel should apply.

_____

_____

_____

_____

_____

_____

_____

_____

_____

_____

_____

_____

C. You are alone in the office, the doctor having been suddenly called away. Describe briefly how you would handle each of the following emergencies.

1. A man comes into the office saying that something has blown in his eye and he is in severe pain.

_____

_____

_____

_____

_____

_____

_____

_____

_____

_____

_____

_____

2. A woman patient from whom you have just drawn a blood sample, suddenly says she feels faint and slumps in her chair.

_____

_____

_____

_____

_____

_____

3. A patient calls, frantically asking what to do for his wife who has apparently taken an overdose of medication. She remains conscious and is not convulsing.

_____

_____

_____

_____

_____

_____

_____

4. A patient telephones seeking help with a nosebleed which has continued for half an hour. The patient has applied pressure.

_____

_____

_____

_____

_____

_____

_____

_____

_____

_____

_____

_____

D. Write in your own words the steps you would take to administer artificial respiration by the mouth-to-mouth method.

_____

_____

_____

_____

_____

_____

_____

_____

_____

_____

_____

_____

E. Describe in your own words the first aid procedure for dislodging a foreign body in the throat when the victim is unable to speak, but is conscious.

_____

_____

_____

_____

_____

_____

_____

F. List four actions which should **not** be taken when faced with a childbirth
    emergency.

    1. _____

    2. _____

    3. _____

    4. _____

    _____

    _____

CHAPTER 6

PLANNING AND KEEPING THE OFFICE

A. 1. List four factors to be considered in estimating the seating requirements for a physician's reception room.

1. Scheduled length of appointment

2. Frequency of times doctor is delayed at hospital or for an emergency

3. Frequency doctor spends more time than planned with patient

4. Percentage of patients who must be accompanied by someone else (Pediatrics, geriatrics, etc)

2. Name eight housekeeping procedures that the medical assistant should check daily to be sure that they have been done properly.

1. Empty waste baskets & reline with disposable bags

2. Wash Countertops and tops worktables & desks

3. Wash lavatories, sinks, toilets, tile

4. Dust all furnishings including bookshelves

5. Vacuum Carpets & spot clean if needed

6. Vacuum furniture & spot clean if needed

7. Clean mirrors & picture frames

8. Clean window coverings - blinds, curtains, drapes

3. List four things that a medical assistant should do periodically during the day in order to keep the reception area in good order.

1. _Doormat in proper position_
2. _Coat hangers in good supply_
3. _Lighting & ventilation comfortable_
4. _Magazines straightened on tables_
   Clean wastepaper baskets
   Clean coffee area

4. Name two things that might have to be prohibited in a reception room in order to avoid harm to certain patients.

1. _Smoking_
2. _Fresh plants or flowers_

5. The file on each major piece of office or medical equipment should include certain items. List five.

1. _Installation & maintenance instruction_
2. _Warranty - Serial #_
3. _Record of service & part replacement_
4. _Name, number & address of supply company_
5. _Name, number & address of repair company_

6. List at least ten items of administrative supplies that you feel would be needed in a typical doctor's office. Include some items not mentioned in Chapter 6 of the text.

1. _Stationery_
2. _Prescription Blanks_
3. _Calling cards_
4. _Insurance forms_
5. _Charge slips_
6. _Medical History forms_
7. _File Folders_
8. _Computer Supplies_
9. _Pens - Pencils - Erasers_
10. _Bill & ledgers_
11. _Duplicating paper_
12.
13.
14.
15.
16.

7. List at least ten items of medical supplies that you feel would be needed in a typical doctor's office. Include some items not mentioned in Chapter 6 of the text.

1. Medications
2. Bandages
3. Cotton
4. Thermometers
5. Syringes
6. Tongue depressors
7. Alcohol
8. Disposable gloves
9. Adhesive
10. Needles
11.
12.
13.
14.
15.
16.

8. List three types of equipment that will minimize odors.

1. Chemicals in spray or liquid form
2. Solid deodorants
3. Electrostatic air cleaner

9. Describe two precautions that might be taken to avoid the loss of prescription blanks.

1. Secure locks on office
2. Never left where patient can reach them.

10. List at least 10 items that might ordinarily be carried in the doctor's bag. Indicate whether they belong under the heading of instruments, medication, or accessories.

INSTRUMENTS	MEDICATIONS	ACCESSORIES
Syringes + needles	Adrenalin	Cotton
Scalpel	Demerol	Bandages
Thermometers	Antibiotic	Prescription Pad
Stethoscope	Eardrops	Sterile Gloves
Scissors	Eyedrops	Specimen Containers

11. What duties does the medical assistant have in regard to the doctor's bag?

(1) Check list to make sure everything doctor wants is in bag
(2) Everything kept in perfect condition
(3) Bag ready at all times —
(4) After doctor returns - check for specimens to lab or refrigerator
(5) Remove & destroy disposable items
(6) Replace & refill used items

12. List the rules regarding the handling of keys to the office.

1. Keys only to personnel who open or close office
2. Keys should not be left where they can be picked up
3. If keys lost - locks should be changed immediately

13. If you were asked to develop a "fire plan" for your office, list four preparations that you would make.

1. Telephone numbers of fire dept & police attached to all phones
2. Fire extinguishers kept in working condition
3. Knowledge of all exits - fire escapes - fire doors
4. Records saved if time to remove -

PRACTICE AND PROJECTS

A. 1. A patient has just left the examining room. Describe what you would do before another patient enters.

Remove all soiled linen - used instruments
Remove used medication - clean tables &
Counter tops with antiseptic - No stains of any
kind - dressing area, lavatory, toilet wiped clean

34

2. How would you remove the following stains?

(1) Blood on your uniform. _Sponge with cool water –_
if not removed – Sponge with alcohol or hydrogen
peroxide and wash with soap & water –

(2) Grease on patient's dress. _Wash with benzine, ether_
or Commercial cleaning fluid –

(3) X-ray developer on the doctor's lab coat. _Dampen with water –_
Apply iodine with dropper to stain until it turns black –
Sponge with x-ray fixer until stain disappears

. You are asked to estimate seating requirements for a reception room for a solo practice pediatrician who schedules appointments at 20-minute intervals. Describe your calculations.

There would be 6 patients in 2 hours –
One patient in 3 is accompanied by some one else –
Therefore it would require a minimum of 8 Seats

. Your doctor has asked you to go through the office and check all rooms to see that they are as free of safety hazards as possible. List five types of hazards to look for.

1. _Rugs & doormats should not have turned up edges_
2. _Wires should not be laid across floor (cover with rug or tape)_
3. _Electrical wires & connections checked for fraying_
4. _Non slip coatings on non carpeted floors_
5. _Sharp edges and corners on furnishings should be avoided_

. Solve the following problems:

1. Disposable hypodermic syringes cost $50 per 100. If they are purchased in quantities of 1,000 or more, the manufacturer allows a discount of 10%.

750 syringes would cost $ _375 –_ or _50_ ¢ each

1,500 syringes would cost $ _675 –_ or _45_ ¢ each

2. If the doctor uses 250 syringes a month, how much would he save a year by making a single purchase for a year's supply rather than 12 single purchase

$ 150

3. At a usage rate of 250 syringes per month, how frequently could you place an order and still obtain the 10% discount?

every 4 months

E. In ordering the following 10 types of medication, indicate at what level of remaining stock an order should be placed and whether you can take advantage of the best quantity price. The pharmaceutical supplier assures delivery within a week of order placement.

TYPE OF MEDICATION	UNITS USED PER MONTH	USUAL EXPIRATION DATE AFTER DELIVERY	ORDER QUANTITY FOR LOWEST UNIT PRICE	LEVEL OF STOCK AT WHICH ORDER SHOULD BE PLACED	SHOULD ORDER BE FOR BEST PRICE QUANTITY (YES OR NO)
A	12	1 year	100	*90 - beginning of 8th month*	*Yes*
B	100	1 year	500	*100 beginning of 5th month*	*Yes*
C	2	1 year	45	*1 beginning of 15th month*	*no*
D	4	18 months	100	*2*	*no*
E	200	2 years	1000	*200*	*Yes*
F	16	6 months	144	*8*	*No*
G	16	1 year	144	*15*	*Yes*
H	20	1 year	144	*20*	*Yes*
I	20	2 years	750	*10*	*No*
J	100	20 months	1500	*100*	*Yes*

F. Make a rough sketch of the floor plan of a doctor's office with which you are familiar and list three or four features that are either desirable or undesirable based on your own judgment of how a doctor's office should be planned.

CHAPTER 7

THE MEDICAL ASSISTANT AS RECEPTIONIST

Complete the following sentences or answer the questions in the blank spaces provided.

1. The first contact that a patient has with a doctor's office is often with the medical assistant who has the job of _receptionist_ .

2. In offices that are open during designated hours and do not have an appointment system, patients are usually seen in order of _appearance ^arrival_ .

3. The space for each entry in an appointment book should be big enough for both the patient's name and _abreviated notation of reason for appt._ (—phone #)

4. If a patient's name is not clear on the telephone, the medical assistant should _ask patient to spell name._ .

5. When a period of fasting is necessary prior to an examination or diagnostic test, the patient's appointment is usually at what time of day? _early AM_

6. Telephone calls from patients about their bills can usually be handled by the _medical assistant_ .

7. Are most doctors likely to have their medical assistants answer the office telephone? _Yes_

8. In making telephone connections, it usually is the courteous thing for the party _initiating_ the call to do any waiting that may be involved.

9. An office telephone call director usually will be located on the _front (receptionist's)_ desk.

10. It is important to keep telephone calls to or from a doctor's office as brief as possible so that *Emergency Calls do not have to wait* .

B. From the items listed under each statement or question, select the correct answer or answers. Write the corresponding letter or letters in the answer space.

1. To plan the best utilization of various office facilities, the medical assistant-receptionist should:

   a. call all patients the day before their appointments as a reminder.
   b. know what rooms, equipment, and personnel will be required for each appointment.
   c. schedule only one complete physical examination per day.
   d. overschedule in the expectation of having some cancellations. *A-B*

2. Which of the following features make for an efficient appointment book?

   a. A type of binding that allows the pages to lie flat on a desk top.
   b. A system for showing what appointment times are filled for an entire week.
   c. Room enough in each appointment space to show the patient's address.
   d. A separate book for each doctor. *A-B*

3. When there is no urgency about the time for an appointment, it is acceptable practice to:

   a. offer the next open date or ask the patient for his or her preference.
   b. suggest a date several weeks beyond the next open date.
   c. suggest an early hour as these times are the hardest to fill.
   d. offer a date when you have only a few appointments. *A*

4. When a patient calls to cancel an appointment, the medical assistant should:

   a. ask the patient the reason for cancelling.
   b. be courteous and set up a new appointment.
   c. suggest that the patient might want to reconsider in view of the difficulty in getting appointments.
   d. point out to the patient that a cancellation charge will be made. *A? B*

5. Which of the following are good practice in greeting a patient entering the office?

   a. Finish any work in process before turning to the patient.
   b. Have in mind the names of the patients that are expected and call them by name.
   c. Interrupt a phone conversation to speak to an incoming patient.
   d. Avoid any conversation that does not relate to the appointment.
   e. If work with other patients permits, give full attention to greeting the incoming patient. *B-E*

6. The selection of reading material for the reception room should:

   a. reflect the doctor's interests.
   b. be mostly health-related magazines.
   c. reflect the medical assistant's interests.
   d. include a variety of subject matter.

   D

7. When a patient is late for an appointment:

   a. see all other patients first, making the late patient wait until last.
   b. inform the late patient that the schedule has been upset by the delay.
   c. proceed with the next patient if he or she is present.
   d. cancel the patient for that day and arrange a subsequent appointment.
   e. try to fit the patient in, provided the doctor has time and other patients will not be inconvenienced.

   C - E

8. When the schedule is delayed because a patient requires more time than is scheduled, the medical assistant should:

   a. try to make up the time on the other patients.
   b. advise the doctor that others are waiting.
   c. explain the delay to the remaining patients.
   d. move some appointments to another day.

   A - (C) - D

9. When the schedule is delayed because the doctor is late, the medical assistant should:

   a. reschedule all patients.
   b. explain the reason for the delay to the patients.
   c. reschedule those patients who do not wish to wait.
   d. simply inform the patients that the doctor is expected momentarily.

   B - C

10. When a patient's incoming telephone call is transferred to the doctor, the medical assistant should:

    a. make out a telephone message slip.
    b. remain on the line for possible instructions from the doctor.
    c. quickly hand the patient's file to the doctor.
    d. request that the patient be brief.

    A - C

11. Which of the following information would be appropriate to include in a Patient Information Folder?

    a. Office hours.
    b. Doctor's medical specialty or specialties.
    c. Policy regarding payment.
    d. Policy regarding participation in Blue Shield and accepting assignment on Medicare claims.
    e. Whom to contact in case of emergency.

    A - B - C - D - E

C. 1. Name six duties of a typical receptionist.

1. Making appointments

2. Obtaining info from patient + originating records

3. Looking after patient while they are waiting

4. Keeping the schedule.

5. Handling telephone calls

6. Filing records - Insurance forms

Billing Patient

2. What are the first and second things to determine when a patient telephones for an appointment?

1. If it is an emergency or can wait reasonable time (name correct)

2. How long office visit will be needed (muchtime)

3. When scheduling a patient for hospitalization, what basic information about the patient would the medical assistant give to the hospital?

Patient's full name   Accomodation desired.

Address   Admitting diagnosis

Telephone number   if ambulance is needed

4. Answer the questions about the following three forms.

a. Appointment Card

(1) When is it used?

Set up patient's next visit

(2) What does it show?

Patient's name - date of next visit

time of next visit

b. Doctor's Calendar

(1) How often is it filled in? Once a day

(2) Where is it kept? On his desk.

(3) What does it show?

Complete list of appointment for the day

(4) From what source is the doctor's appointment information taken?

Appointment book

c. Use of Equipment Schedule

(1) What does it show?

Date, time, name patient, Doctor
Time each patient is scheduled to use each piece of equipment

(2) What is the source of this information?

Appointment book

5. List two types of telephone calls that usually are handled independently by the medical assistant.

1. _Appointments (Patients)_

2. _Calls from pharmaceutical representatives_
Insurance inquiries

PRACTICE AND PROJECTS

A. Make a list of the magazines you would recommend for the reception room of a Gynecologist-Obstetrician.

Childbirth
New Mothers
Women's Magazines on all subjects

B. Your doctor's policy is to see patients by appointment. Briefly describe what you would do if a patient came into your office without an appointment.

Determine if it is an emergency - if yes - fit in patient as soon as possible - if not fit in if an opening exists - if no opening - reschedule for available time

C. If you were working for a solo practitioner and he or she were suddenly taken ill, expecting to be confined to bed at home for several days, what would you do about the patients scheduled for those days?

Call & explain situation (with doctor's permission)
if prompt medical attention is needed —
refer to other doctors —
(Have patient call directly)

If absence unexpected — call standby
physicians to see if they can take
patients temporarily.

D. Your doctor-employer has designated the hours of 8:30 to 9:30 a.m. as the time when he will receive telephone calls from patients. One of your regular patients calls at 10:00 a.m. How would you handle the situation?

Check if emergency —
if not, take message and relay to
doctor at first opportunity.
Make up call slip and tell patient
doctor will return call asap — Give
message to doctor along with patient's file.

E. Fill out the registration slip pictured on the following page as if you were the patient. Add notes at the bottom regarding your preferences for appointment times and where you wish to be contacted by telephone.

REGISTRATION SLIP

PLEASE PRINT   DATE _8/9/9?_

NAME _BARBARA LEWIS_

ADDRESS _22 S. BAYARD LANE_

CITY _MAHWAH, NJ_   ZIP CODE _07430_

Telephone _327-3567_   Birth Date _9/9/_   Sex _F_

☐ Single   ☑ Married   ☐ Widowed   ☐ Divorced

Occupation _RETAILER_   Phone _930-0949_

Employed by _YOUNG ELEGANCE_

Employer's address _WOODCLIFF LAKE, NJ_

Name of Spouse _SAMUEL_

Occupation _RETAILER_   Phone _930-0949_

Employed by _SAME_

Employer's address _____

Referred by _____

INSURANCE: Soc. Sec. Number _131-26-9105_

Medical Insurance Cert. No. _____

Company _BLUE CROSS/BLUE SHIELD_

Hospital Insurance Cert. No. _SAME_

Company _____

Other Health Insurance _AARP_

_23540465_

FORM NO. 3320, COLWELL CO., CHAMPAIGN, ILL.

CALL 930-0949 - NO APPTS TUESDAY

F. A patient, who has not been to the office for several months, calls and asks to speak to the doctor giving no indication that there is an emergency. How would you respond in order to try to handle the call independently?

check if patient is ill. Try to get more information about symptoms. If emergency and doctor is not busy, buzz to see if he wants to speak to patient. If doctor busy, get all info possible, and tell caller doctor will get back as soon as possible. Make out complete call slip - attach patient's file and give to doctor.

G. A patient calls and clearly has an emergency. The doctor is in but is examinin
another patient. What should the medical assistant do?

_Be sure it really is an emergency —
Remain calm & composed — Tell caller to
stay on line and connect with doctor at once.
If doctor not in, get name, address, phone # plus_ *

H. You have received the three telephone messages given below. Write out a
memorandum to Dr. Brown about each one. Use the forms on page 43. What, if
anything, would you attach to the memoranda?

_① Patient's Records — ② Patient's records ③ Dr's insurance file
if available_

1. Mrs. Margaret O'Dwyer calls at 9:10 a.m. to say that she had abdominal pain
and a slight fever. You have told her that Dr. Brown is not in the office
but is expected shortly and that you will ask him to call her as soon as he
comes in. The registration file shows that Mrs. O'Dwyer lives in East
Hills; telephone 555-0123.

2. Mr. William Curtis calls at 9:15 a.m. to say that he has to leave town that
evening and will have to cancel his appointment for the following day. He
would like to know whether it will be all right to skip the injection
scheduled or whether he should stop at the office late today. He asks that
Dr. Brown call him as soon as possible at his office, 555-1123.

3. Mr. Sidney Harman of the Prudential Insurance Company calls at 9:30 a.m.
He wishes to discuss the doctor's insurance program, as he feels it needs
bringing up to date. He will call back on the following day for an
appointment.

*_ name of nearest emergency medical unit if caller
knows, Look up unit number, put caller
on hold and notify emergency unit —
Notify call, unit on way and give
first-aid instructions if able to carry them out,
Call back in 15 min to check on caller._

44

Phone Message

TO
☑ LOCAL ☐ LONG DISTANCE

M_Mrs. Margaret O'Dwyer_

of _East Hills_

Telephoned	✓	Call him/her		Returned your call	
Came in		Will call you			

PHONE 555-0123

MESSAGE:
abdominal pain
slight fever

Taken by _BR_ Date _8/7/92_ Time _9:10_ a.m./p.m.

Phone Message

TO
☑ LOCAL ☐ LONG DISTANCE

M_r. Sidney Furman_

of _Prudential Insurance Co._

Telephoned	✓	Call him/her		Returned your call	
Came in		Will call you	✓		

PHONE

MESSAGE: Will call for
appointment to update
insurance program

Taken by _BR_ Date _8/7/92_ Time _9:30_ a.m./p.m.

Phone Message

TO
☑ LOCAL ☐ LONG DISTANCE

M_r. William Curtis_

of

Telephoned	✓	Call him/her		Returned your call	
Came in		Will call you			

PHONE 555-1123

MESSAGE: has to leave town +
cancelled appt for tomorrow
Is it all right to skip
injection scheduled or
should he stop by office
late today?

Taken by _BR_ Date _8/7/92_ Time _9:15_ a.m./p.m.

45

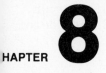

THE MEDICAL ASSISTANT AS SECRETARY

UIZ

From the items listed under each question, select the correct answer or answers. Write the corresponding letter or letters in the answer space.

1. If a letter (received or sent out) deals with several patients:

   a. the required number of copies are made and a copy filed in the folder of each patient.
   b. the letter is filed in the folder of the first patient mentioned.
   c. cross-references are made for the second and third patient mentioned and filed in their respective folders.
   d. the letter is filed in the folder of any one of the three patients discussed. _____

2. Numeric filing is used when:

   a. there are too many folders for each letter of the alphabet.
   b. anonymity of the patient is desired.
   c. filing is done by the rotary method.
   d. alphabetizing is too complicated. _____

3. In a doctor's office, patients' histories are usually filed:

   a. in active, inactive, and closed files.
   b. in vertical, rotary, and visible systems.
   c. by subject and alphabetically.
   d. according to their diseases. _____

4. Membership in medical societies:

   a. increases the doctor's practice.
   b. furnishes him with malpractice insurance.
   c. usually includes subscriptions to the society's publications.
   d. offers the possibility of making friends among doctors. _____

5. When the doctor is not available to sign a letter and the assistant is authorized to do so, the assistant should:

   a. sign the doctor's name by copying his handwriting as closely as possible.
   b. sign the letter by printing the doctor's name.
   c. omit the signature.
   d. write the doctor's name followed by the assistant's initials. _____

6. You are Dr. Alan B. Smith's secretary and your name is Mary Louise Brown. What would be acceptable ways to show initials at the bottom of the doctor's letters?

a. ABS:mlb   e. ABS/mlb
b. abs:mlb   f. abs:mlb
c. ABS-mb   g. mlb
d. ABS:mb

                                                     _____

7. When using window envelopes, addresses on bills should be positioned as follows:

a. in the center of the bill head.
b. so that the full address can be read by shifting the bill within the sealed envelope.
c. so that the full address will show through the window no matter how much the bill shifts within the envelope.
d. so that a minimum space of 1/8" shows around the full address no matter how much the bill shifts within the envelope.   _____

B. 1. What type of spacing should be used between lines of letters?

_____

2. What are two methods of paragraphing most commonly used in letter writing?

1. _____

2. _____

3. What two practices can be followed to be certain that the reader will have no doubt about a date in a letter?

1. _____

2. _____

4. Pages following the first page of a letter should show what information at the top of the page?

_____

5. How do you find a paper quickly that may be filed under more than one name or subject?

_____

_____

6. Name the three basic systems of sequential order used in filing.

1. _____

2. _____

3. _____

7. How are prefixes such as von, O', or Mc treated in filing names alphabetically?

_____

8. What determines the sequence when filing correspondence of persons with the same surname?

_____

9. Are such titles as Dr., Mrs., Colonel considered in alphabetic filing?

_____

10. How would you file a reprint?

_____

11. When writing a letter to the office of a group of three doctors whose names are Smith, Brown, and Jones, how would you write the salutation?

_____

12. What type of spacing between lines is usually used in addressing envelopes?

_____

13. What are the standard two-letter abbreviations for your state and each of the other states that border on your state?

_____

14. If your doctor-employer received a copy of an article written by another doctor, would you consider it good secretarial performance to type up an acknowledgment and give it to your doctor for signature along with the article?

_____

15. Name three types of secretarial duties that a medical assistant may be asked to perform that do not directly pertain to the operation of a medical office.

1. _____

_____

2. _____

_____

3. _____

_____

16. List four characteristics of paper (other than size) that you would want to consider in selecting stationery for the office.

    1. _____   3. _____

    2. _____   4. _____

17. What part of an address should be within an envelope's OCR (Optical Character Recognition) area in order to facilitate automatic handling by the Postal Service?

    _____

18. The OCR (Optical Character Recognition) area of an envelope may be described as an imaginary rectangle that has:

    its top _____ inches up from the bottom of the envelope.

    its bottom _____ inches up from the bottom of the envelope.

    its sides _____ inch in from the sides of the envelope.

19. The "Bar Code Area" of an envelope is a 4½-inch long, 5/8-inch high strip located in what part of an envelope?

    _____

20. Name the major bibliographical index to medical literature and the issuing organization.

    _____

    _____

21. List five subjects that might be covered in an Office Policy Manual under the subject of EMPLOYMENT POLICIES.

    1. _____

    2. _____

    3. _____

    4. _____

    5. _____

    _____

    _____

The following is a copy of a Library of Congress index card. From this material, find the answers to the questions following it.

Duncan, Garfield George, 1901–   *ed.*
   Diseases of metabolism : detailed methods of diagnosis and treatment. Edited by Garfield G. Duncan. 5th ed. Philadelphia, W. B. Saunders Co., 1964.
       xxii, 1551 p. illus. (part col.) 26 cm.
   Includes bibliographies.

   1. Metabolism, Disorders of.   I. Title.

RB147.D8   1964   616.39   64–10654

   Library of Congress   [7–1]

1. Is Mr. Duncan the author?_____

2. Who is the publisher? _____

3. Under what subject would you file this card? _____

4. What edition is this? _____

5. How many pages are in the book—exclusive of introductory pages? _____

6. What is the copyright date? _____

PRACTICE AND PROJECTS

1. Your doctor-employer has been asked by Dr. John Allen, Chairman of the local AMA program committee, to serve on that committee. Your doctor asks you to write a letter explaining that he is unable to serve now because he expects to leave shortly on a ten-week trip, but would like to serve later. Compose the text of the letter.

   _____

   _____

   _____

   _____

   _____

   _____

   _____

   _____

   _____

2. Write a letter dated November 25, 1985, to Dr. Joseph E. Brown of White Clinic, Newton, Massachusetts 02666, asking whether your doctor's patient, Mrs. Mary Green of 35 Orchard Street, Oldtown, Rhode Island 02555, had kept an appointment on November 5, 1985, as no report has been received from the clinic and the patient has not been in touch with our office. Your doctor's name is Susan J. White.

3. While on vacation in another state, Wilma R. Weber, a patient, suffered temporary amnesia and was hospitalized from November 8 through 11, 1985. She is now recovered, back home, and was in to the office on November 25, 1985. Your doctor, Susan J. White, would like to have the hospital records. Write the appropriate letter. The hospital is City General Hospital, Front Street, Benton, Massachusetts 02707. Mrs. Weber's address is 140 Orchard Street, Oldtown, RI 02555.

_____

_____

_____

_____

_____

_____

_____

_____

_____

_____

_____

_____

_____

_____

_____

_____

_____

_____

B. Indicate the alphabetic order of the following names by writing the correct sequence number before each name.

1. _____ D'Andries, Emile

2. _____ Mayberry, Laura

3. _____ McMillan, Margaret

4. _____ Sabel, Maude

5. _____ Yoest, Hans

6. _____ Zelnig, Gretchen A.

7. _____ Walker, Carl J.

8. _____ Van Dusen, Maureen

9. _____ St. Clair, Ethan

10. _____ Margolis, John

11. _____ Ochman, Gerald

12. _____ Capt. Lear, Mortimer S.

13. _____ DeCarlo, Jan D.

14. _____ Dana, Elbert

15. _____ Abbott, Allen A.

16. _____ LeMay, Cortland

17. _____ Newmann, Janice

18. _____ Walker, A. J.

19. _____ Zellig, Edmund

20. _____ Vance, Reed D.

21. _____ Madden, Elsie

22. _____ Lea, Olive

23. _____ Danato, Angelo

24. _____ MacElroy, Joseph

25. _____ Sanders, Edna R.

26. _____ Abbott, Alma (Mrs. Albert A.)

27. _____ Lemont, Leland

28. _____ Walker, Adrienne J. (Mrs. Carl J.

29. _____ Connor, Donald D.

30. _____ MacKenzie, Donald R.

31. _____ Prof. Veneble, Vance

32. _____ MacBirney, Coleen

33. _____ Rev. Dow, B. V.

34. _____ Clair, I. D.

35. _____ Col. Yost, O. J.

36. _____ O'Connor, Julia

37. _____ Davis, June

38. _____ McKenzie, Mary J.

39. _____ MacKenzie, Ralph A.

40. _____ Abbott, Alan J.

41. _____ Dowd, Alice

42. _____ Newman, James

43. _____ Dr. Saunders, B. R.

44. _____ Mace, Genevieve

45. _____ McElroy, Roy

46. _____ Debold, Ethelbert

FFICE MAIL

{Z

Complete the following sentences or answer the questions using the blank spaces.

1. In general, doctors will expect the details of a satisfactory mail-processing system to be worked out by _The medical Assistant_ .

2. By what time after its arrival in the office should mail be routed to the person who will handle it? _As early in the day as possible_

3. Persons sending mail to the office will expect it to be looked at on the day _it is received_ .

4. Would a letter addressed to the doctor and marked confidential generally be given to the doctor unopened? _Yes_

5. Would the medical assistant who opens the incoming mail be expected to scan the contents and decide to whom in the office the items should go? _Yes_

6. Checks received in the mail should be endorsed in what manner to insure that no one else can cash them if they are lost or stolen? _endorsed for bank deposit only_

7. How frequently should outgoing mail be posted? _At least once a day before last pickup_

8. First-class mail is more confidential because _it may not be opened without a federal search warrant_ .

9. The most reliable and safest form of mail delivery is _first class registered_ .

10. What should be done about the office mail when the office will be closed on a normal mail-delivery day? _Arrangements should be made with mail carrier to hold mail until next day._

11. Addresses on packages should be in large enough lettering so that the address is readable at about what distance? *Arms length*

12. What are the minimum length and height of an envelope that will be accept by the Postal Service? _____*5"*_____ length; ___*3½"*___ height

13. When the office is to be moved, how much notice should be given to the Po Office? *few days*; patients? *at least a month*

14. When you are notifying a magazine publisher of a change of address, cut the *mailing label* from an old issue of the magazine and paste it

in the "old address" space on the Change of Address card.

B. From the items listed under each question or statement, select the correct answer or answers. Write the corresponding letter or letters in the answer space.

1. If your mail carrier's schedule is to deliver to the office in midafterno what other arrangements might be made to assure earlier delivery?

   a. Request special carrier service.
   b. Schedule your working hours later.
   c. Allow time in your afternoon schedule for adequate handling of the normal mail.
   d. Rent a post-office box and pick up mail in early morning. *C D*

2. When an incoming letter, which will be placed on the doctor's desk, refers to prior correspondence, the medical assistant should:

   a. give this mail priority.
   b. give this mail routine timing.
   c. attach prior correspondence to the current letter.
   d. hold the letter aside for later discussion with the doctor. *C*

3. Postage meters may be advantageous in a doctor's office:

   a. when the office is mailing numerous parcels of different size.
   b. in order to save on postage.
   c. in order not to run short of postage.
   d. to eliminate the need for post-office cancellation. *A X-?*

4. Mailgrams are appropriate to use when:

   a. the message is short.
   b. it is desirable to have the message in writing.
   c. delivery is desired the following day.
   d. All of the above. *D*

5. The advantage of a postal money order is that it:

   a. does not deplete the office cash.
   b. has the immediate value of cash.
   c. has the equivalent of a bank guarantee.
   d. is as safe to mail as a check.

   B - D   C?

6. If the doctor rents a post office lockbox, when would it be possible to pick up mail there?

   a. Anytime
   b. Daily except Sundays and holidays
   c. Whenever the lobby of that particular post office is open
   d. Every day on which there is mail delivery service

   ~~D~~ C

7. Which of the following package wrapping materials are preferred by the Postal Service?

   a. Masking tape
   b. Self-adhering tape with filament reinforcement
   c. Wrapping paper and strong twine
   d. Strong twine without wrapping paper

   B

8. In addressing packages, which of the following are proper procedure?

   a. Show both destination address and return address on only one side of the package.
   b. Show destination address on both sides of the package.
   c. Enclose a separate sheet of paper within the package showing address, return address, and description of contents.
   d. Show ZIP codes on a separate final line.

   A - C

9. In 9-digit ZIP codes, the last 4 digits are used to identify

   a. small parts of a postal route, such as one side of a city block.
   b. individual residences.
   c. a particular mail carrier's route.
   d. mail which can only be handled with automated sorters.

   A

10. The bar codes on letters

    a. permit automatic sorting of letters into the individual locations recognized in 9-digit ZIP codes.
    b. are applied by the Postal Service.
    c. identify the sender's location.
    d. are designed to be read by automatic sorting equipment.

    ~~ABC~~ - D

C. 1. List six types of incoming mail that would be routed to the doctor.

1. Reports from testing laboratories on patients.
2. Patients correspondence requiring doctors attention
3. Bills for major expenditures - business correspondence for doctor
4. Notices from professional organizations
5. Professional journals, flyers
6. Announcements concerning medications, office supplies, etc.

2. List at least seven types of incoming mail that the medical assistant usually would handle.

1. Payments - checks or cash
2. Insurance forms (routine)
3. Letters from patient not requiring doctor (routine)
4. Magazines for office
5. Bills for routine office supplies & services
6. Catalogs not related to medicine
7. Change of address notices
8. Returned mail
9.

3. A patient writes to the doctor complaining about the type of treatment received and inability to get a satisfactory explanation.

a. Would you route this letter to the doctor for handling? Yes

b. What would you attach to such a letter for the doctor's full information on the case?

Patients file and correspondence

58

4. When outgoing mail is picked up from a central collection point in the office, what things should the medical assistant be sure are done before this material is posted?

Correct postage applied
Return address showing
Wrapping and sealing properly done
Special marking if required ("Fragile" - "Do not fold")

5. List two types of special mailing containers frequently used by doctors.

1. _X-rays (need stiff cardboard backing)_
2. _For blood and lab samples to testing laboratories_
   Fiberboard boxes

PRACTICE AND PROJECTS

. You are opening the morning mail and find $25 cash in one envelope, but nothing else. The envelope shows the name and return address of one of the doctor's patients. What would be your immediate action?

_____

_____

_____

_____

_____

. A note from a patient states that $20 is being paid on account but only one $10 bill is found in the envelope. What action would you take?

_____

_____

_____

_____

_____

_____

C. Visit your local post office and obtain pamphlets explaining the full range of
    current services. List the types of service you believe would be used by a
    group practice of three doctors. The office occasionally requires next-day
    delivery and mails x-ray films and written material of an individual nature
    weighing over 12 ounces.

    _____

    _____

    _____

D. Your solo doctor-employer is attending a two-week international conference out
    of the country. What action would you take in the following two instances?

    1. A letter is received from a patient complaining about the amount of a bill
        and demanding an immediate answer.

        _____

        _____

    2. A patient requests certain records be sent to her immediately so they can
        be taken to an out-of-town clinic.

        _____

        _____

E. During your visit to the local post office, mail a first-class letter and obtain
    a "Certificate of Mailing." Fill out the certificate, present it with the letter
    to the postal clerk, have the certificate stamped by the clerk and pay the fee.

    _____

    _____

    _____

CHAPTER 10

PATIENTS' RECORDS

UIZ

. From the items listed under each question or statement, select the correct answer or answers. Write the corresponding letter or letters in the answer space.

1. Information from a patient's record should not be released to a third party unless:
    a. the patient asks that the information be released.
    b. written authorization for release is signed by the patient.
    c. the patient's employer arranged for the patient's examination.
    d. it is information pertaining to an insurance examination.   _B_

2. Medical ethics require the doctor to:
    a. treat all information about the patient as confidential.
    b. provide medical information about a patient to other doctors who request the information.
    c. inform health officials of cases of communicable diseases.
    d. provide patients with a reasonable standard of care.   A-B-C-D

3. Telephone calls from patients concerning treatment:
    a. need not be entered into the patients' records.
    b. should be noted by the assistant on the record.
    c. should be noted on the record including date, significant comments from patient, and doctor's response.
    d. should be noted in the appointment book.   B-C

4. X-ray films are considered to be:
    a. the property of the patient.
    b. the property of the physician.
    c. part of the medical record.
    d. as confidential as any other medical data about the patient.   B-C-D

5. When taking any part of the medical history, the assistant should:
    a. seat the patient in as private an area as possible.
    b. make notes of relevant facts the patient may mention.
    c. avoid the possibility that other persons may overhear the questioning.
    d. allow a third party to be present if the patient requests.   A-B-C-D

6. Which of the following represent good practice in filing patients' medical records?
   a. The files of patients' medical records should be kept separate from other office files.
   b. The records of children of the same parents may be filed in a common file jacket.
   c. X-rays that are too large for standard size file cabinets may be kept in separate cabinets that are of sufficient size.
   d. The cabinets holding patient records should be lockable.

   A-C-D

7. Which of the following steps might you take to keep the number of patients' records files within reasonable and efficient limits?
   a. Transfer files of patients who have not been seen for about two years into an "inactive" file.
   b. Transfer files of patients who are deceased into a "closed" file.
   c. Transfer files of patients who change to another physician to a "closed" file.
   d. Microfilm old files for which the doctor wants to retain a record.

   A-B-C-

8. "Problem Oriented Records" refer to a system of keeping patients' medical records which:
   a. classifies patients according to major physical problem.
   b. records the diagnosis, treatment, and outcome of each of a patient's medical problems in a separate sub-section of the patient's total record.
   c. is regarded as probably providing more concentrated attention on each separate medical problem a patient might have.
   d. is directed exclusively to problems of a strictly medical nature.

   B-C

B. 1. List below the main purpose of patients' records and two additional purposes.
   Main purpose: *Provide doctor with all significant information accumulated to date so doctor can best judge how to proceed*

   Additional purposes:

   1. *Source for doctor to provide synopsis of case to send to another physician.*

   2. *Important legally. Support patient claim for personal injury or protect doctor against charge of malpractice.*

62

2. Name seven types of information that would be found in a patient's record in addition to the patient's history.

1. _Findings of the physical exam. - ~~Allergies~~_
2. _Laboratory test results_
3. _X-rays, electrocardiograms, other tests_
4. _Records and evaluations from other doctors_
5. _Copies of hospital records for inpatient or outpatient services_
6. _Doctors summary, impressions, instructions or treatment of patient_
7. _Correspondence with patient or about patient concerning medical matters -_

3. Classify the following information in a patient's record as either subjective or objective.

1. Patient's complaints   _Subjective_
2. Urinalysis   _Objective_
3. Patient's family history   _Subjective_
4. Patient's list of past illnesses   _Subjective_
5. Patient's habits   _Subjective_
6. Spleen not palpable   _Objective_
7. Menstrual cycle   _Subjective_ ~~_Objective_~~
8. Normal cervix   _Objective_
9. Temperature, pulse, and respiration   _Objective_
10. Patient's identification of letters in an eye examination   _Subjective_

4. Name six kinds of "personal habits" that might be covered in a medical history.

1. _Smoking_
2. _Drinking_
3. _Drugs - medical or recreational_
4. _Exercise_
5. _Occupation_
6. _Sexual activities_

63

5. List two advantages of shelf filing for patients' records.

1. _When file in use shelves open leaving all jackets on shelves open to view_

2. _Shelves roll out allowing for top & side access to jackets –_

6. List two ways in which color coding of the tabs of file jackets would make a more efficient filing system for patients' records.

1. _Guides user to small section of files for faster accessibility_

2. _Reduces misfiling –_

7. SOAP is an acronym that represents a logical series of steps a doctor would take in dealing with any medical case. What do each of the letters stand for?

1. "S" _Subjective data (patient's symptoms)_

2. "O" _Objective data (doctors exam + findings)_

3. "A" _Assessment (diagnosis)_

4. "P" _Plan of action (treatment_

8. The computer in your office is used primarily for financial records but has some excess capacity to store a limited amount of medical data about each patient. Suggest one item of medical information that might be added to the data in the computer for each patient and briefly describe how such information might be used.

Medication for patients taken on regular basis.

If medication was found to have harmful side effects, doctor could contact patient for further study & analysis or to change medication.

PRACTICE AND PROJECTS

A. The information below was entered on a patient's record. On May 20 it was discovered that the patient was in the office on May 16 instead of May 17 and that the patient's hemoglobin was incorrectly recorded as 16 g when it should have been 14 g. What would you do about the record?

May 16, 1985—Pain much relieved; symptoms subsiding; discomfort only after

fatty foods. BP 140/90; P 86; HB 16 g.

On examination, abdomen slightly tender. Continue medication

until prescription finished. Recheck in one month.

B. Study the two medical records given below. Transfer the information to the forms provided. The date is November 5, 1985.

1. The patient's name is John Andrews; date of birth 9/30/76. His father is Frederic Andrews, and they live at 51 West 3rd Street, Anytown, KS 67XXX. Telephone 555-1111. They were referred by Dr. W. G. Smith, phone 555-1122.
    The child complained of sore throat and chills since yesterday. His temperature was 101°, pulse 120, respiration 25. Only significant findings were enlarged, beefy tonsils. Blood count showed hemoglobin 16; white blood cell count 11,000 with 76% polymorphonuclears, 16% large lymphocytes, 6% monocytes and 2% small lymphocytes. Urine normal. Throat culture taken.
    Tentative diagnosis: acute tonsillitis, nonfollicular. Prescribed children's aspirin, 2 tabs. q 4 hrs. pending culture results. Father to call tomorrow for report of culture.

2. The patient's name is Arnold Boots, aged 36. His address is 420 E. 21st Street, Beetown, IL 60XXX; telephone 555-0012. He was referred by Mrs. Gale and he is a salesman and single.
    His father is 62, his mother 58, and they are both living and well. A sister is also alive and well. There are no significant diseases in the family.
    The patient had measles at age 6, and mumps at 10; only surgery a tonsillectomy at age 19. He uses alcohol minimally; smokes about ½ pack of cigarettes per day; has normal appetite; no previous indigestion; bowel movements regular and normal; no recent strenuous activity.
    He complains of chills, severe pain in the abdomen. Examination showed marked tenderness in the right lower quadrant, over the McBurney point.
    He is 5'8" tall and weighs 172 pounds. Temperature 102°, pulse 100; respiration 20; BP 120/76. Chest sounds normal; lungs clear; no rales; heart regular.
    CBC showed 20,000 total white blood cell count with 88% polymorphonuclears, 10% lymphocytes, 1% monocytes.
    A diagnosis of acute appendicitis was made, and immediate hospitalization was ordered.

B.1

CASE NO. _____ PATIENT'S NAME _____

ADDRESS _____ INSURANCE_____ DATE_____

TEL. NO._____ REFERRED BY _____ AGE_____ SEX_____

FAMILY HISTORY: PARENTS:_____

   CHILDREN LIVING_____DEAD_____CAUSE_____ MISCARRIAGES_____CAUSE_____

INFANT HISTORY: DATE OF BIRTH_____FULL TERM_____WEIGHT_____BREAST FED_____WHY WEANED_____

   WALKED_____TALKED_____TOXOID_____VACCINATED_____SHICKED_____DICKED_____PERT. VAC._____SCAR. FEVER_____TYPH._____T. B._____

   TYPE OF FEEDING: FREQUENCY_____QUANTITY_____KIND _____

   APPETITE_____COLIC _____CONSTIPATION_____NUTRITION _____

   VOMITING _____STOOLS_____

PRESENT ILLNESS: DURATION_____SYMPTOMS _____ONSET_____

   PAIN _____COUGH_____FEVER_____CRY_____SLEEP_____APPETITE_____VOMIT_____STOOLS_____ERUPTIONS _____

PHYSICAL EXAMINATION: WEIGHT_____HEIGHT_____HEAD_____EYES_____EARS_____TEETH_____GUMS_____THROAT_____

   TONSILS_____ADENOIDS _____FONTANEL_____BACK _____NECK_____GLANDS_____LUNGS_____HEART_____

   ABDOMEN_____SKIN_____SPLEEN_____LIVER_____EXTREMITIES _____GENITALIA_____NERVOUS SYSTEM_____

LABORATORY FINDINGS:_____

DIAGNOSIS:_____

TREATMENT: _____

REMARKS:

HISTACOUNT®   PEDIATRICS FORM NO. 1160   HISTACOUNT CORPORATION, MELVILLE, L. I., N. Y.

B.2

CASE NO. _____ PATIENT'S NAME _____

ADDRESS_____ INSURANCE_____ DATE_____

TEL. NO._____ REFERRED BY _____ OCCUPATION_____ AGE_____ SEX_____ S. M. W. D.

FAMILY HISTORY_____
_____
_____

PAST HISTORY_____
_____
_____

PRESENT AILMENT_____
_____
_____

PHYSICAL EXAMINATION: TEMP._____PULSE_____RESP._____B. P._____HEIGHT_____WEIGHT_____

   SKIN_____MUCOUS MEMBRANE_____EYES_____EARS_____NOSE_____MOUTH_____

   NECK_____CHEST _____LUNGS_____HEART_____ABDOMEN_____RECTUM_____

   VAGINA_____GENITALS_____EXTREMITIES_____OTHER_____

LABORATORY FINDINGS:_____

DIAGNOSIS:_____

TREATMENT: _____

REMARKS:_____

HISTACOUNT®   GENERAL PRACTICE FORM NO. 1150   HISTACOUNT CORPORATION, MELVILLE, L. I., N. Y.

CHAPTER 11

FEES, BILLS, CREDIT, AND COLLECTIONS

QUIZ

A. From the items listed under each statement or question, select the correct answer or answers. Write the corresponding letter or letters in the answer space.

1. Fee schedules are:
   a. a price list a doctor prepares to show what the charges are for each of the more common services.
   b. prepared by the local Blue Shield organization.
   c. dated to indicate the period when the prices shown are effective.
   d. the basis for quoting fees to patients.   *A-C-D*

2. In discussing the fee with the patient, the medical assistant should:
   a. express regret regarding fees patients feel are high.
   b. tell the patient that fees will be determined after treatment is completed.
   c. under no circumstances quote a definite fee.
   d. quote the fee according to the doctor's instructions.   *D*

3. Which of the following are economic factors that influence the level of fees a doctor establishes for individual services?
   a. Office costs, such as rent and utilities
   b. The fees charged by other doctors offering similar services in the same community
   c. Employee salaries
   d. The doctor's family budget   *A-B-C-D*

4. Which of the following are acceptable procedures for charge slips?
   a. Doctor keeps supply of charge slips, marks services performed; medical assistant fills in fees.
   b. Medical assistant writes patient name and date on charge slip, attaches it to patient file; doctor fills in services performed and fees.
   c. Doctor initiates charge slips, attaches each one to the patient's record and places in outbox for pickup by medical assistant later in the day.
   d. Charge slips should be numbered as a means of ensuring all patients' visits are accounted for.   *A-B-D*

5. As a means of encouraging patients to pay at the time of each office visit, the assistant might:
    a. total the charge slip the patient turns in and ask if he or she would care to pay now.
    b. ask the patient for payment prior to seeing the doctor.
    c. post a sign indicating that payment is expected with each visit.
    d. offer a premium for each payment.   A - C

6. When patients pay at the time of each visit:
    a. it is not necessary to fill out a ledger card for the patient.
    b. it is not necessary to send a monthly bill.
    c. a receipt should be given.
    d. a monthly bill should be sent showing charge and payment.   B - C

7. Patient ledger cards may be posted from the following sources:
    a. charge slips.
    b. the daily record.
    c. invoices from outside laboratories.
    d. records of payments from patients.   A - B - D

8. Patient ledger cards show the following information:
    a. outstanding balances owed by the patient.
    b. collection fees.
    c. payments made by the patient.
    d. charges made to the patient.
    e. the services performed for each charge.   A - C - D - E

9. "Cycle billing" refers to:
    a. sending bills at uniform intervals, such as monthly, weekly, or twice a month.
    b. sending bills to all patients at the end of each month.
    c. sending bills as soon as possible after each office visit.
    d. grouping charges by type of service instead of date.
    e. sending bills for groups of accounts, one group every so many days.   E

10. It is good practice to itemize bills:
    a. to avoid mistakes in figuring the total amount.
    b. to show patients and insurers the amount charged for each service.
    c. to make it easier for patients when preparing their income tax reports.
    d. to give the doctor a detailed listing of services performed for each patient.   A - B - D

11. When a patient pays a bill in cash:
    a. the payment should be entered on the ledger card.
    b. a statement showing payment should be sent promptly.
    c. a receipt should be given or sent to the patient.
    d. the patient should be sent a note of thanks.   A - C

68

12. Superbills typically include more information than appears on other types of bills used by doctors. Which of the following are examples of such additional information?
    a. The insurance company's codes for procedures the doctor has performed.
    b. The diagnosis.
    c. Space for the patient to authorize release of information.
    d. Date of next appointment.
    e. Doctor's signature.   *A - B - C - D - E*

13. Bills owed by patients who have died should be sent to:
    a. the patient's home address in his or her name.
    b. the executor of the deceased patient's estate.
    c. the deceased patient's lawyer.
    d. the nearest living relative.   *B*

14. Telephone conversations with patients regarding overdue bills should be:
    a. courteous, unemotional, and considerate of patients' financial difficulties.
    b. firm in asserting the doctor's need for the funds.
    c. apologetic regarding the size of the bill.
    d. limited to the person responsible for payment.   *A - D*

15. Which of the following responses should be made if the patient is worried about the size of the bill?
    a. The doctor's fees, once quoted, will not be changed.
    b. The doctor's fees are in line with what others charge.
    c. A method can be worked out to spread the cost over a period of time.
    d. The doctor's fees are reasonable compared to others.   *C*

16. Which of the following statements are correct?
    a. Misunderstandings about bills are less likely if the doctor's charges are discussed in advance.
    b. Patients expect a discount if they pay in cash.
    c. Insurers require itemized bills.
    d. Doctors' offices sometimes use computerized billing services.   *A - C - D*

17. Which of the following are advantages of a "pegboard" system of keeping business records?
    a. Less chance of discrepancies among the various business records of the office.
    b. Several basic business records are produced in one writing.
    c. Patients will be less concerned about the accuracy of their bills.
    d. Insurance claims will be paid more promptly.   *A - B*

18. Which of the following are legal obligations of the doctor in deciding whether to extend credit to a particular patient?
    a. The amount of payment per month must be scaled to the patient's income.
    b. Other creditors of the patient must not be contacted to determine the patient's record for paying bills.
    c. The patient may not be refused credit simply because he or she is receiving public assistance.
    d. If a credit report on the patient is unfavorable, the doctor must identify the credit agency to the patient.   *C - D*

69

19. What should the assistant be sure to do to prepare for making a telephone call to a patient who is delinquent in paying a bill?
    a. Check the patient's credit rating in the local credit bureau.
    b. Verify the exact amount owed and for how long.
    c. Check with the doctor to see if the bill may be reduced.
    d. Check to see what the patient may have promised in any previous telephone call.

    B - D

20. When an overdue account is turned over to a collection agency:
    a. the patient's ledger card should be so noted.
    b. subsequent payments received from the patient should be forwarded to the agency.
    c. the doctor may consider that medical obligations to the patient have ended.
    d. the doctor should be certain that he or she still has the right to cancel the debt.

    A - B - D

21. In a "preferred provider organization":
    a. the term "provider" refers to participating doctors or hospitals.
    b. the providers are preferred because of their reputation for high quality service.
    c. the charges to participating patients would be higher than those to other patients.
    d. participating insurers typically pay all of a medical bill.

    A - D

22. What response should an assistant make when a patient indicates inability to pay a bill in one payment?
    a. Try to get a definite commitment for payment of a definite amount per month.
    b. Indicate that the bill may be given to a collection agency.
    c. Offer to settle for a portion of the total bill.
    d. Agree to postpone the due date until the full amount can be paid.

    A

B. Answer the following questions in the space provided. Be specific.

1. Name at least three types of individuals that may be treated free of charge or given a professional discount by the doctor.

    1. *Clery*
    2. *Health Care Professionals (nurses, doctors, dentists)*
    3. *Family members of doctors*

70

2. Name five forms that may be used to prepare bills.

   1. _Charge slips_
   2. _Receipt book_
   3. _Ledger cards_
   4. _Daily record sheets_
   5. _Superbill_

   _____

3. During the past year, insurance claims covering your doctor's charges for a urinalysis have shown that the regular fees were $10 on ten claims, $12 on ten claims, and $15 on ten claims. For the current year, what would Blue Shield's calculation be for the doctor's:

   "usual charge" for a urinalysis? _$15 (75%)_

   "profile charge" for a urinalysis? _doctor's usual charge $15 (90%)_

4. Define "customary charges" as used in the Blue Shield UCR program.

   90th percentile of the usual fees charged by doctors in same specialty in same general area for given procedure

5. Under Medicare Part B, what is the doctor agreeing to when he or she "accepts assignment"?

   doctor agreed amt, approved under Medicare rules will be payment in full.

6. In a Medicare Part B claim, the doctor's regular fee is $50. Medicare approves a charge of $40. The patient has satisfied all but $10 of the deductible for the current year. The doctor accepts assignment.

   1. What amount is paid by Medicare? _$24_

   2. What amount may the doctor bill the patient? _$16_

   3. What is the total amount received by the doctor? _$40_

   _____

   _____

7. Should a ledger card be made for:

   cash patients? _Yes_   free patients? _Yes_

   patients receiving professional discounts? _Yes_

8. Ledger cards that are to be photocopied to make bills require certain information that is not needed on ledger cards that are used for internal office purposes only. List two items of such information that should appear on the ledger cards for photocopying.

1. _Patient's name + address (heading) positioned to fit window envelope_

2. _Bottom section looks like bill_
   Payment expected in so many days

_____

9. List four business office forms that would be incorporated in a typical "pegboard" system.

1. _Charge slips_   2. _Daily record_

3. _Ledger cards_   4. _receipt_

10. What two conditions make a doctor's credit agreement with a patient subject to the "Truth in Lending Act"?

If finance charges are added

If payment is more than 4 installment

When either or both of these conditions prevail:

(1) Must the agreement be in writing? _Yes_

(2) How must any finance charges be expressed? _As an annual rate_

Is it the position of the American Medical Association that doctors should not charge interest on credit accounts?

Yes

PRACTICE AND PROJECTS

A. Compose a brief collection letter from Dr. Green to Mr. Brown, a patient who has been owing $165 for four months in spite of two reminders. You may use a typed letterhead or the space below.

B. The following entries appear in your daily journal for new patients.

DATE	NAME	SERVICE	CHARGE	PAID
June 2	Jose Gonzalez	Office visit	$25	$25 (check)
	Werner Rostock	Examination	50	
		X-rays	40	
		Laboratory tests	25	
3	Giselle Morton	Injection	15	10 (cash)
	Jose Gonzalez	ECG	35	
4	Werner Rostock	Physical therapy	20	
6	Giselle Morton	Injection	15	20 (cash)
8	Werner Rostock	Physical therapy	20	115 (check)
	Jose Gonzalez	Office visit	25	

Use the forms provided, as follows:

1. Transfer these entries to the patients' ledger cards (two kinds of ledger forms are provided. Patient's name is typed in.)

2. Make out a receipt for Giselle Morton's cash payment of June 3.

3. Complete the charge slip as it would look for Mr. Rostock on June 2.

4. Make out bills for Jose Gonzalez and Werner Rostock for the period June 1 through June 8. Use the traditional statement forms provided. Assume no prior balances. List all charges first, then payments, and last the balance due.

1.

ALVIN MYLES JONES, M. D.

965 WALT WHITMAN ROAD

MELVILLE, N. Y. 11746

HAMILTON 1-1200

Jose Gonzales

DATE	PROFESSIONAL SERVICE	CHARGE	PAID	BALANCE

CASE NO.   Gonzales, Jose   NAME

Pay Last Amount In Balance Column

OC - OFFICE CALL   HCD - HOUSE CALL DAY   S - SURGERY
HV - HOSPITAL VISIT   HCN - HOUSE CALL NIGHT   BC - BLOOD COUNT
OB - OBSTETRICAL   BMR - BASAL METABOLISM   X - X-RAY
LAB - LABORATORY   EKG - ELECTROCARDIOGRAM   NC - NO CHARGE

ALVIN MYLES JONES, M. D.

965 WALT WHITMAN ROAD

MELVILLE, N. Y. 11746

HAMILTON 1-1200

Giselle Morton

DATE	PROFESSIONAL SERVICE	CHARGE	PAID	BALANCE

CASE NO.   Morton, Giselle   NAME

Pay Last Amount In Balance Column

OC - OFFICE CALL   HCD - HOUSE CALL DAY   S - SURGERY
HV - HOSPITAL VISIT   HCN - HOUSE CALL NIGHT   BC - BLOOD COUNT
OB - OBSTETRICAL   BMR - BASAL METABOLISM   X - X-RAY
LAB - LABORATORY   EKG - ELECTROCARDIOGRAM   NC - NO CHARGE

74

1.

Werner Rostock

DATE	PROFESSIONAL SERVICE	CHARGE	PAID	BALANCE

Pay Last Amount In Balance Column ⬆

2.

No. 3520	No. 3520	Date _____
Date _____	Received of _____	
Name _____	_____	
_____	for professional services	ALVIN MYLES JONES M.D. 965 Walt Whitman Road Melville, N. Y. 11746
_____		
Amount _____	Payment _____	
Balance _____	Balance _____	By: _____

3.

No. 2732   DATE_____

PATIENT'S NAME___Werner Rostock_____

ADDRESS_____

SERVICES RENDERED	FEE	√
CONSULTATION–EXAMINATION		
X-RAY		
INJECTION		
SURGERY		
DIATHERMY		
LABORATORY		
DRUGS		
TOTAL		

NEXT APPOINTMENT_____

PLEASE LEAVE WITH RECEPTIONIST

4.

STATEMENT

ALVIN MYLES JONES, M. D.
965 Walt Whitman Road
Melville, N. Y.   11746
421-1200

_____ 19____

For Professional Services:

STATEMENT

ALVIN MYLES JONES, M. D.
965 Walt Whitman Road
Melville, N. Y.   11746
421-1200

_____ 19____

For Professional Services:

C. 1. Prepare a coded bill (using the form below) for Gunnar Swenson, 2222 Main Street, Champaign, IL 61820. The bill should include a night visit on November 9 for $50.00; 2 house visits during the day on November 10 and 11 at $35.00 each; an office visit at $25.00, ECG at $40.00, x-rays at $48.00, and lab tests at $28.00, all on November 15; and an office visit on November 20 at $25.00. Mr. Swenson paid $120.00 on account on November 15.

STATEMENT

LEONARD S. TAYLOR, M.D.
2100 WEST PARK AVENUE
CHAMPAIGN, ILLINOIS 61820

TELEPHONE 367-6671

Gunnar Swenson
2222 Main Street
Champaign, Il 61820

DATE	PROFESSIONAL SERVICE	CHARGE	PAID	BALANCE
Nov 9	NIGHT VISIT	50 —		50 —
Nov 10	HOUSE VISIT	35 —		85 —
Nov 11	HOUSE VISIT	35 —		120 —
Nov 15	OFFICE VISIT	25 —		145 —
Nov 15	ECG	40 —		185 —
Nov 15	X RAYS	48 —		233 —
Nov 15	LAB TESTS	28 —		261 —
Nov 15	PAYMENT		120 —	141 —
Nov 20	OFFICE VISIT	25 —		166 —

1603

PAY LAST AMOUNT IN THIS COLUMN

OC - OFFICE CALL
HC - HOUSE CALL
HOSP - HOSPITAL CARE
L - LABORATORY
I - INJECTION

INS - INSURANCE
OB - OBSTETRICAL CARE
PAP - PAPANICOLAOU TEST
OS - OFFICE SURGERY
HS - HOSPITAL SURGERY

PE - PHYSICAL EXAMINATION
EKG - ELECTROCARDIOGRAM
XR - X-RAY
M - MEDICATION
NC - NO CHARGE

78

2. Complete the charge slip Dr. Taylor would make out on November 15.

No. 2801

DATE _____

PATIENT'S NAME   Gunnar Swenson

ADDRESS _____

SERVICES RENDERED	FEE
EXAMINATION	
OFFICE VISIT	
X-RAY	
INJECTION	
SURGERY	
DIATHERMY	
LABORATORY	
ECG	
TOTAL	

NEXT APPOINTMENT _____

PLEASE LEAVE WITH RECEPTIONIST

. On June 30, you survey the ledger cards in your office and find that three patients have not paid their bills for several months. Bills are sent out on the last day of each month; the doctor expects payment within 30 days of billing and considers that two months after billing the account is 30 days past due.

Patient A had charges of $50 in January and nothing has been received or charged since.

Patient B had charges of $100 in February; paid $50 in March; had charges of $25 in March; and no further entries in the account.

Patient C had charges of $80 in November; paid $40 in April; had charges of $60 in May; and no further entries in the account.

Fill in the following analysis form.

PATIENT	TOTAL AMOUNT PAST DUE	DAYS OVERDUE - AMOUNT				
		30	60	90	120	OVER 120

ACCOUNTS RECEIVABLE AGING ANALYSIS AS OF JUNE 30

PATIENT	TOTAL AMOUNT PAST DUE	30	60	90	120	OVER 120
A	$					
B						
C						

HE DOCTOR'S ACCOUNTS
—MANUAL AND
COMPUTERIZED

UIZ

.. From the items listed under each question, select the correct answer or answers. Write the corresponding letter or letters in the answer space.

1. The record in which office expenses are kept is called:
   a. the patient's ledger.
   b. the general ledger.
   c. the daily journal.
   d. record of office disbursements.   _D_

2. The daily record would include charges made by the doctor for:
   a. hospital calls.
   b. home visits.
   c. consultations.
   d. office services.   _A-B-C-D_

3. The term petty cash refers to:
   a. bills and coins on hand to make change when patients pay cash.
   b. coins listed for bank deposits.
   c. a cash fund kept on hand for small expenditures.
   d. all cash receipts not entered in the daily journal..   _A-C_

4. The daily record of receipts should include:
   a. receipts received when paying office expenses.
   b. checks received in the mail from patients.
   c. cash received from patients.
   d. checks received in payment of insurance claims.   _B-C-D_

5. The patients' ledger cards are:
   a. records of charges to and receipts from each patient.
   b. equivalent to the doctor's accounts receivable.
   c. part of the patients' medical records.
   d. posted from charge slips in some instances.   _A-B-D_

6. Which of the following expenses would be entered in the Record of Disbursements?
   a. The amount of an employee's total salary prior to withholdings for social security or income tax.
   b. Expenses for use in the doctor's home.
   c. Purchases of medications that will be dispensed to patients in the office.
   d. A check to be cashed to replenish the petty cash account.   _C-D_

7. The amount of cash generally used to set up a petty-cash fund is:
    a. $20.
    b. $50.
    c. $100.
    d. based on the expected minor cash expenditures for a month.   ~~B~~ D

8. To replenish the petty cash a check is drawn for:
    a. the original amount.
    b. the amount spent.
    c. the amount estimated for the next month's expenses.
    d. whatever is adequate to meet current expenses.   B

9. To prove the accuracy of the petty-cash account at any time:
    a. the money on hand is totaled and compared with the
        original amount.
    b. the checks drawn for petty cash are added up.
    c. the daily items under Disbursements are added up.
    d. expenditures from the fund and cash on hand are totaled
        and compared with the original amount.   D

10. The income tax that the doctor must withhold from the medical
     assistant:
    a. is an amount agreed to by the assistant.
    b. is a certain percent of the assistant's salary.
    c. depends on the number of withholding allowances and amount
        of the salary.
    d. equals one-twelfth of the estimated annual tax.   ~~A~~-C-~~D~~

11. The amount of pay posted in the Disbursement Record for an employee is:
    a. the net pay check after all deductions.
    b. the regular monthly salary for the employee.
    c. the full hourly earnings for the employee.
    d. all of the above.   A -

12. Which of the following statements are correct?
    a. The employee pays all the social security tax applicable
        to an employee's wage or salary.
    b. An unmarried person age 30 with no dependents would
        generally claim one allowance on a W-4 form.
    c. There is no social security tax on earnings of part-time
        employees.
    d. An employee's state and local income taxes may be withheld
        by the employer.   B-D

13. Which of the following statements are correct?
    a. Both the federal government and state governments have
        unemployment compensation taxes.
    b. In most states the rate of unemployment compensation taxes
        varies depending on the employer's record for providing
        stable employment.
    c. Both federal and state unemployment compensation taxes
        have maximum amounts of individual employee earnings to
        which the taxes apply.
    d. Payments of state unemployment compensation taxes are
        made quarterly.   A-B-C-D

14. "Workers' Compensation" refers to:
    a. wages paid on an hourly basis.
    b. wages or salaries paid to employees.
    c. state required insurance programs that must be carried by
       employers in order to provide benefits to employees who
       are injured or contract diseases on the job.
    d. self-employment earnings.

    C

15. Which of the following functions might a computer perform
    in a doctor's office?
    a. Fill out insurance claim forms.
    b. Print billing statements.
    c. Make out charge slips.
    d. Complete consent forms.
    e. Prepare a payroll.

    A - B - ~~C~~ - E

16. In a computer system that handles the financial information
    in the office, which of the following would be sources of
    information which the medical assistant would enter into
    the computer?
    a. Duplicates of receipts for cash or checks received from
       patients in the office.
    b. Telephone calls from patients inquiring about bills.
    c. Charge slips.
    d. Bills ready for mailing to patients.

    A - C - ~~D~~

17. Which of the following would be correct with regard to a
    computer system in a doctor's office?
    a. A letter-quality printer would provide a lesser quality
       of printing than dot matrix.
    b. CRTs should be faced away from the reception area.
    c. It is preferable to have more than one person in an
       office familiar with the operation of the computer.
    d. A 256K computer would not necessarily have more
       memory capacity than a 64K unit.

    B - C

18. In double entry bookkeeping which of the following would be
    correct?
    a. Cash or check received is entered as a debit to cash.
    b. A charge to the patient for services rendered is entered
       as a credit.
    c. When a patient pays for only part of the total charges
       for services, the unpaid balance is entered as a debit
       to "Accounts Receivable."
    d. A check paid out is entered as a credit to cash.
    e. A check paid out is entered as a debit to cash.
    f. A trial balance is a summation of all debit entries and
       a summation of all credit entries to see if the two
       totals agree.

    A - B - C - D - F

B. 1. List seven basic records which make up a doctor's financial accounts.

1. Daily record of charges + receipt + monthly summary
2. Individual patient ledger cards
3. Record of office disbursements
4. Employment records
5. Petty cash account
6. Summary records of charges, receipts + office disbursement (for quarter or year)
7. Checkbook + bank statements

2. When the medical assistant keeps the daily record (or journal) the information for posting to the record will come from several sources. Name three.

1. Charge slips + records of visits at home or in hospital
2. Duplicates of receipts given for payment in cash or check
3. Checks received in mail from patient or insurance companies

3. List two types of withholdings that must be made from employee salaries und[er] Federal law.

1. FICA - Federal Insurance Contribution Act (Social Security)
2. FIT - Federal Income Tax

4. What items make up the difference between the balance on a bank statement and the balance in the checkbook?

1. deposits not on statement
2. Checks not cancelled
3. service charges

5. Describe three checks for accuracy that might be made in the Daily Record o[f] Charges and Receipts.

1. Balance ledgers
2. Check invoices for accuracy
3.

6. When the bank returns a check for insufficient funds, describe what you would do.

   Contact patient immedeately (if for insufficient funds), tactfully explain situation and ask if check can be redeposited. Redeposit on separate deposit slip with explanation - Correct checkbook balance.

7. What is meant by a cash discount?

   Discount given for payment within a very short period of time (usually 10 - 30 days)

8. What financial information shows on the W-2 form?

   1. Gross amount of salary for year
   2. Amounts withheld for FICA, FIT
   3. Amounts withheld for State & local taxes
   4. Net salary
   5. Ins. or other deductions

9. How often is a complete statement of withholdings of social security and income taxes sent to the Internal Revenue Service?

   Quarterly

10. Are unemployment compensation taxes in most states withheld from employees or paid entirely by the employer?

    Withheld from employees

11. How should checks be identified on deposit slips?

    By American Bankers Association number (Stamped on back with endorsement "For deposit only in account of Dr — Acct #)

12. Name three types of employment benefit programs that a doctor might have f
his or her employees.

1. *Group hospitalization & medical insurance plan*
2. *Life insurance on employee*
3. *Pension plans*

13. Under an accrual system of accounting, on what dates would the following
transactions be recorded as income to the doctor?

(1) Patient treated on October 20; pays before
leaving office. *Oct 20th*

(2) Patient treated on October 20; bill sent to
patient October 31; patient pays bill on
November 5. *Oct 20th*

(3) Patient treated on October 20; doctor files
claim with Blue Shield on October 22; Blue
Shield sends check to doctor on November 20. *Oct 20th*

14. What are the four main pieces of computer hardware that would typically be
required in a doctor's office?

1. *keyboard including 10-key numerical pad & function keys*
2. *video screen similar to TV screen - show info entered*
3. *Central processor - stores information*
4. *Printer - automatically types output*

PRACTICE AND PROJECTS

A. The entries listed below represent the doctor's charges and receipts for one
day, September 15, 19XX.

1. Enter each item on the daily record page provided.

2. Make out a deposit slip for the cash and checks received. The doctor's
name is Roy Clark, M.D. His account number is 037 1 18149 in City Guaranty
Trust Company.

3. The sum of the cash and check receipts on the Daily Record should be the
same as the total of the deposit slip. If not, you have made an error; go
over your entries and addition.

NAME	SERVICE	CHARGES	RECEIPTS
George Morton	Office visit	$ 35	$ 45 check (Union Bank)
Waldemar Bachmann	Office visit	35	
	Injection	20	20 cash
Inez Gonzalez	Office visit	35	35 cash
Irving Levy			25 check by mail (Peoples Bank)
Franz Steckel	ECG	40	75 check (Peoples Bank)
Margaret Hunter	Lab tests	55	30 cash
Walter O'Neill	X-rays	28	
	Medication	15	43 cash
John Cabot			120 check by mail (City Guaranty Trust)
Sandra Godinski			65 check by mail (Union Bank)
Anne Taylor	Office visit	30	30 cash

The ABA codes are:

Union Bank   1-23/567   Peoples Bank   1-8/567   City Guaranty Trust   1-10/567

1. On the days indicated, the following disbursements were made, all by check. Enter each one on the Disbursement page in the appropriate columns on the form provided.

DATE	NAME	DISBURSEMENT	
Sept. 1	Rosen Real Estate Co.	$ 1700.00	rent
4	New York Telephone Co.	245.47	
4	Consolidated Light Co.	227.00	
14	City tax collector	320.00	
15	American X-ray Company	180.00	repairs
15	Mildred Warner	657.50	semimonthly paycheck
23	Anchor Service Station	81.11	gasoline
24	Plaza Pharmaceuticals	156.88	drugs
30	Gordon Pollock, CPA	300.00	accountant's fee
30	North American Instrument Co.	187.65	ECG electrodes
30	American College of Physicians	150.00	dues
30	Mildred Warner	657.50	semimonthly paycheck

2. Prepare checks for the doctor's signature for September 15 on the forms provided; post the September 15 bank deposit in the checkbook. The doctor's checkbook balance at the end of September 14 was $1500.50.

3. The doctor asks you for the checkbook balance at the end of September 15.

   What is the amount?_____

DAILY RECORD OF CHARGES AND RECEIPTS

DATE —

PATIENT	CHARGES	RECEIPTS		OFF. VISIT	CHARGES FOR TYPE OF SERVICE			
		CASH	CHECK		LAB	X-RAY	INJ.& MED	ECG
1								
2								
3								
4								
5								
6								
7								
8								
9								
10								
11								
12								
13								
14								
15								
16								
17								
18								
19								
20								
21								
22								
23								
24								
25								
26								
TOTAL								

REGULAR CHECKING

DEPOSITED IN

City Guaranty Trust Company

ALL DEPOSITS ACCEPTED SUBJECT TO THE CONDITIONS
STATED ON THE REVERSE SIDE OF THIS DEPOSIT SLIP.

	Dollars	Cents
BILLS		
COINS		
CHECKS 1		
2		
3		
4		
5		
6		
7		
8		
9		
10		
11		
12		
13		
14		
TOTAL		

DATE_____

FOR THE ACCOUNT OF

_____
(PLEASE PRINT)

ACCOUNT NUMBER										

RECORD OF OFFICE DISBURSEMENTS

FOR MONTH OF _____

DATE	PAYEE	TOTAL AMOUNT	TYPE OF EXPENSE					
			EMPLOY-MENT	RENT & UTILITIES	MEDICAL SUPPLIES	X-RAY & ECG	AUTO	MISC.

No. *115*	Roy Clark, M. D.	No. *115*

_____ 19 ____

_____

Pay to the
order of

_____ 19 —

$_____

	$	
Bal. forwarded		
Amount dep. Amt. deposited		
Total		
Amt. this check		
Balance		

City Guaranty Trust Co. _____

037-1-18149

No.	Roy Clark, M. D.	No.

_____ 19 ____

_____

Pay to the
order of

_____ 19 —

$_____

	$	
Bal. forwarded		
Amount dep. Amt. deposited		
Total		
Amt. this check		
Balance		

City Guaranty Trust Co. _____

037-1-18149

C. Complete the following employment figures, using social security at 14.10% for employee and employer combined.

1. Monthly payroll

EMPLOYEE	SALARY	SOCIAL SECURITY WITHHELD	FEDERAL INCOME TAX WITHHELD	NET SALARY PAID
"A"	$1500	$ _____	$ 300.00	$ _____
"B"	1200	_____	210.00	_____
"C"	1000	_____	175.00	_____
Total	3700	_____	685.00	_____

2. Employer's Quarterly Tax Return, covering one quarter.

EMPLOYEE	TAXABLE WAGES PAID TO EMPLOYEES DURING QUARTER
"A"	$ _____
"B"	_____
"C"	_____
Total	_____

Total Federal income tax withheld during quarter. . . . _____

Total social security taxes applicable on salaries
paid during quarter . . . . _____
(This report and any prior monthly deposits)

Total amount remitted to IRS for the quarter. . . . . . _____

D. Fill in the following double entry journal and ledger forms for the September 1 transactions involving patients Morton, Bachmann, Gonzalez, and Levy (see Project A) and the disbursements to American X-ray Company and Mildred Warner (see Project B). Assume Mildred Warner's semi-monthly salary is $800 and withholding are $142.50. Also, on the ledger forms, fill in the "debit" and "credit" headings.

After completing the ledger forms, take a trial balance for these entries only.

JOURNAL

Date	Account Titles and Explanation	Debit	Credit	
				1
				2
				3
				4
				5
				6
				7
				8
				9
				10
				11
				12
				13
				14
				15
				16
				17
				18
				19
				20
				21
				22
				23
				24
				25
				26
				27
				28
				29
				30
				31
				32
				33
				34
				35
				36
				37
				38
				39
				40

LEDGER ACCOUNTS

Cash		Accounts Receivable		Accounts Payable

Services Rendered		Expense-X-ray & ECG		Employment

Trial Balance:

    Total Debits   _____

    Total Credits   _____

CHAPTER 13

INSURANCE
FOR THE PATIENT

1. Indicate with a "yes" or "no" whether the following pairs of words belong together.

   1. Overtime—workers' compensation *No*

   2. Insurance—collections

   3. Medicare—Social Security Administration *Yes*

   4. Blue Shield—hospitalization SURGICAL *No*

   5. Blue Cross—surgical fees HOSPITAL *No*

   6. Health insurers—third parties *Yes*

   7. Carriers—insurance organizations handling Medicare
      Part B

2. What steps does the assistant take to identify and record a patient's health insurance coverage?

   1. *Ask for patient's insurance ID card.*
   2. *Enter on registration card or ledger card or*
   3. *Computer base all data on card including name of ins. Carrier, type of coverage, agreement no. and patients group or ID number.*

3. Which of the following are usually covered by Blue Shield?

1. Anesthesiologist's fee? _____ ✓
2. Hospital nursing care? _____
3. Hospital room? _____
4. Surgeon's fee? _____ ✓
5. Diagnostic electrocardiogram? _____ ✓
6. X-ray for broken arm? _____ ✓
7. Routine office visit? _____
8. Annual physical examination? _____
9. Workers' compensation case? _____
10. Diagnostic laboratory tests? _____ ✓

4. Does Medicare medical insurance Part B pay for:

1. Pacemaker? _____ ✓
2. Hearing test for a hearing aid? _____
3. In-patient hospital charges? _____
4. Out-patient hospital charges? _____
5. Diagnostic x-rays in physician's office? _____ ✓
6. X-rays in a routine physical examination? _____ ?
7. In-patient skilled nursing facility charges? _____ ✓
8. Surgeon's fee? _____ ✓
9. Routine eye examination for glasses? _____
10. Medications that cannot be self-administered? _____ ✓
11. Doctor's visit to patient's home? _____ ✓
12. Injection administered by office nurse? _____ ?

5. Your doctor's regular fee for an ECG is $40 and you performed an ECG for diagnostic purposes on the following two patients:

1. A patient with Blue Shield 100 coverage. Your doctor participates in Blue Shield. Blue Shield records show your doctor's "usual" charge for an ECG to be $35 and the "customary" charge to be $34. What would be the charge approved for payment by Blue Shield? $ 35

2. A Medicare patient with Part B coverage. Your doctor accepts assignment. Medicare's approved charge is $30. What is the amount your doctor can accept for an ECG on this patient? $ 24

From whom will the doctor receive the above amount under the following three circumstances?

		AMOUNT FROM MEDICARE	AMOUNT FROM PATIENT
(1)	Patient has had no previous Medicare Part B claims in the year.	$ —	$ 30
(2)	Patient has had previous approved Medicare charges in the year of $200.	$ 24	$ 6
(3)	Patient has had previous approved Medicare charges in the year of $65 (assume Part B deductible is $75).	$ 14	$ 16

3. If your doctor did not accept assignment under Medicare, what amount would be billed to a Medicare patient for an ECG? $ 30

6. An "Explanation of Medicare Benefits" shows the following information about five patients. What amount could the doctor bill the patient in each case?

	APPROVED AMOUNT	AMOUNT APPLIED TO DEDUCTIBLE	CO-INSURANCE	AMOUNT TO BE BILLED TO PATIENT
(1)	$100	$ 0	$ 20	$ 0
(2)	100	75	5	75 -
(3)	100	50	10	50 -
(4)	50	50	0	50 -
(5)	50	0	10	0

From the items listed under each question, select the correct answers. Write the corresponding letter or letters in the answer space.

1. To pay medical expenses of an employee injured on the job, an employer carries:
    a. health insurance.
    b. malpractice insurance.
    c. workers' compensation insurance.
    d. Medicare.   C

2. Under Medicare Part B, the deductible refers to:
    a. the accumulated amount of Medicare approved charges which the patient must pay before Medicare will cover part of any further approved charges.
    b. the accumulated amount of actual charges which the patient must pay before Medicare will cover part of these charges.
    c. 80% of the charges for covered services.
    d. the amount doctors deduct from their regular fees in billing Medicare patients.   A

3. Medicare Part B is:
   a. applicable to all persons eligible for social security at age 65.
   b. available to persons who are eligible for social security at age 65 and who sign up for Medicare medical insurance.
   c. applicable to persons over 65 who do not have private health insurance.
   d. inapplicable to persons in a prepayment plan.   *B-*

4. In Medicare Part B, coinsurance refers to:
   a. the 20% of approved charges Medicare does not pay.
   b. the insurance that is paid by Medicare.
   c. the amount of unapproved charges.
   d. the amount the patient pays for uncovered services.   *A*

5. Blue Cross provides insurance for:
   a. surgeons' fees.
   b. doctors' consultation fees.
   c. hospital charges.
   d. home nursing care.
   e. anesthesiologists' fees.   *C*

6. The types of plans offered by Blue Shield include:
   a. fee-schedule plans.
   b. "usual, customary, and reasonable" plans.
   c. capitation plans.
   d. plans which pay only a percentage of approved charges. *A-B-D*

7. Workers' compensation insurance provides:
   a. income for laborers without jobs.
   b. safe working conditions.
   c. payment of worker's wages while ill.
   d. payment of doctor's bills if worker is injured in the course of employment.   *D*

8. When a doctor does not accept assignment under Medicare:
   a. he nevertheless is limited to his "customary fee".
   b. he is not entitled to any payment.
   c. he will bill the patient directly and the patient files the claim.
   d. he processes the claim for a reduced fee.   *C*

9. If a health-insurance policy has a deductible feature of $100, this means that:
   a. the patient can deduct this amount from the doctor's bill.
   b. the patient has to pay this amount.
   c. the doctor cannot charge more than $100 for any one service.
   d. the insurance company will reimburse the patient for $100 only.   *B*

10. To file an insurance claim it is usually necessary to:
    a. complete a claim form.
    b. send in the x-rays and laboratory reports.
    c. furnish a copy of the patient's medical record.
    d. write out a detailed report.   *A*

11. Which of the following must sign the "Health Insurance Claim Form"?
    a. The doctor performing the service.
    b. A Medicare patient even though the signature may be on file in the doctor's records on a blanket statement.
    c. A Medicare patient who has not signed a blanket statement for the record of the physician performing the service.
    d. A Blue Shield subscriber who is the insured.
    e. A Blue Shield patient.

    A

12. Medicare Part B claims are handled by:
    a. private insurance organizations under contract with the federal government.
    b. the Department of Health, Education, and Welfare.
    c. the social security office.
    d. an insurance company.

    C

13. The Medicare claim number usually is:
    a. the number of the policy.
    b. the patient's social security number with a suffix.
    c. the doctor's case-history number.
    d. a number assigned to each individual on Medicare.

    B

14. Supplies of Medicare claim forms can be obtained from:
    a. the Department of Health, Education, and Welfare.
    b. a stationer.
    c. the National Institutes of Health.
    d. the insurance carrier.
    e. any Social Security office.

    D-E

15. A "Preferred Provider Organization" is one in which:
    a. the physician's charges for serving member patients are usually relatively low.
    b. patients are encouraged to go to the most qualified physicians.
    c. the physician members are limited to serving patients who are participants.
    d. patients are limited to the doctors designated by the insurance carrier.

    A-D

1. List at least six points that are important in completing insurance forms so as to minimize delay in payment of the claim.

    1. *Accuracy + neatness*
    2. *Read instructions and familiar self with form*
    3. *Doctor consulted on med info not clear from patient record*
    4. *Contact ins co. about technicalities*
    5. _____
    6. _____
    7. _____

8. _____

9. _____

10. _____

2. List three things a doctor has agreed to do when he or she is a participating doctor in Blue Shield.

1. _Limit Charges to those approved by B.S._

2. _Submit forms direct to BS for payment_

3. _____

_____

3. List four health-insurance programs that may be classified as tax-supported programs.

1. _Medicare Part A & B_

2. _Medicaid_

3. _CHAMPUS (Dependents of service personnel)_

4. _CHAMPA_

Workers Compensation

4. List two things a doctor agrees to when he or she accepts assignment under Medicare.

1. _Accept amt approved by Medicare as full charge for services_

2. _Doctor submits & prepares claim forms._

PRACTICE AND PROJECTS

A. Prepare a Health Insurance Claim form for patient Mary A. Brown who is the wife of John W. Brown, 246 Eighth Ave., Woodsville, KY 12345, telephone 555-2109. Mrs. Brown was born February 2, 1945. Mr. Brown carries Blue Shield insurance, identification number 802468024, Group number 865; no other health insurance. About the beginning of June, Mrs. Brown began experiencing irregular heart beats, general fatigue, and light-headedness; she made an appointment for June 10, 1986 and was given an ECG ($40) and single chest x-ray ($35). A complete blood count and sedimentation rate were done in the office laboratory ($30 and $15, respectively). There was no previous record of symptoms of this kind. The visit was for intermediate service ($42). Diagnosis was iron-deficiency anemia.

Procedure codes from Blue Shield Procedure Manual (CPT-4 effective 1/1/85):

```
Electrocardiogram, complete      93000
X-ray chest—single view          71010
Office visit, intermediate       90060
CBC                              85031
ESR (Wintrobe)                   85650
```

Your doctor's name is Ben V. Newburg, M.D., 800 Fourth St., Woodsville, KY 12345; telephone 555-2287; social security number 123-45-6789. No payment was received from the patient. The reverse side of the Health Insurance Claim Form indicates that under "Place of Service" the doctor's office is "O". Block 24-G of the form does not need to be filled in for Blue Shield claims.

Prepare a Health Insurance Claim form for patient Amos B. Cadbury, 135 Seventh Ave., Woodsville, KY 12345, telephone 555-3197. Mr. Cadbury was born October 15, 1919, and has Medicare Part B insurance; his Medicare number is 789-10-1112A. About mid-May, Mr. Cadbury began having diarrhea which continued for several weeks along with abdominal pain in the lower left quadrant. He made an appointment for June 8, 1986. Dr. Newburg performed a proctoscopic examination ($50) and a complete blood count ($30) was done. The visit was intermediate. The diagnosis was "Irritable colon". For Medicare claims, the procedure codes are from CPT-4 (Common Procedure Terminology, 4th edition, issued by the American Medical Association, effective 1/1/85).

```
Applicable codes are:  Proctoscopy                  45300
                       CBC                          85031
                       Office visit, intermediate   90060
```

Mr. Cadbury had no similar symptoms previously; he carries no other health insurance. He has made no payment to the doctor. For block 24-G on the insurance form a code on the reverse side of the form is as follows:

```
        1—Medical care (includes proctoscopy and office visit)
        5—Diagnostic laboratory
```

Your doctor, William W. Wheat, M.D., does not accept assignment under Medicare but your duties include filling out medicare claims for patients to send to the insurance carriers. Fill in a Patients' Request for Medicare Payment form for Joseph P. Jones, 791 Ninth St., Townville, PA 56789, telephone 717-555-4321, medicare number 345-67-8910A. Mr. Jones came to the office complaining of palpitations and shortness of breath. He has a history of hypertension. Mr. Jones was given an ECG and chest x-ray—2 views—and was diagnosed as having cardiomegaly (enlarged heart). Mr. Jones is not employed and is not covered by other medical insurance.

You should also make sure that Mr. Jones has a bill from Dr. Wheat itemizing the ECG, chest x-rays, and office visit. Notice that the claim form was pre-printed to show the address of the insurance carrier to which the claim should be mailed by the patient. Most offices will have forms that show the carrier's address for the area. Caution the patient to sign and date the form and attach itemized bills.

HEALTH INSURANCE CLAIM FORM

(CHECK APPLICABLE PROGRAM BLOCK BELOW)

| ☐ MEDICARE (MEDICARE NO.) | ☐ MEDICAID (MEDICAID NO.) | ☐ CHAMPUS (SPONSOR'S SSN) | ☐ CHAMPVA (VA FILE NO.) | ☐ FECA BLACK LUNG (SSN) | ☐ OTHER (CERTIFICATE SSN) |

PATIENT AND INSURED (SUBSCRIBER) INFORMATION

1. PATIENT'S NAME (LAST NAME, FIRST NAME, MIDDLE INITIAL)

2. PATIENT'S DATE OF BIRTH

3. INSURED'S NAME (LAST NAME, FIRST NAME, MIDDLE INITIAL)

4. PATIENT'S ADDRESS (STREET, CITY, STATE, ZIP CODE)

5. PATIENT'S SEX MALE ☐ FEMALE ☐

6. INSURED'S ID NO. (FOR PROGRAM CHECKED ABOVE, INCLUDE ALL LETTERS)

7. PATIENT'S RELATIONSHIP TO INSURED SELF SPOUSE CHILD OTHER

8. INSURED'S GROUP NO. (OR GROUP NAME OR FECA CLAIM NO.)
☐ INSURED IS EMPLOYED AND COVERED BY EMPLOYER HEALTH PLAN

9. OTHER HEALTH INSURANCE COVERAGE (ENTER NAME OR POLICYHOLDER AND PLAN NAME AND ADDRESS AND POLICY OR MEDICAL ASSISTANCE NUMBER)

10. WAS CONDITION RELATED TO

A. PATIENT'S EMPLOYMENT YES ☐ NO ☐

B. ACCIDENT AUTO ☐ OTHER ☐

11. INSURED'S ADDRESS (STREET, CITY, STATE, ZIP CODE)

TELEPHONE NO.

11.a. CHAMPUS SPONSOR'S

STATUS: ☐ ACTIVE DUTY ☐ RETIRED ☐ DECEASED BRANCH OF SERVICE

12. PATIENT'S OR AUTHORIZED PERSON'S SIGNATURE (READ BACK BEFORE SIGNING)

I AUTHORIZE THE RELEASE OF ANY MEDICAL INFORMATION NECESSARY TO PROCESS THIS CLAIM I ALSO REQUEST PAYMENT OF GOVERNMENT BENEFITS EITHER TO MYSELF OR TO THE PARTY WHO ACCEPTS ASSIGNMENT BELOW

SIGNED   DATE

13. I AUTHORIZE PAYMENT OF MEDICAL BENEFITS TO UNDERSIGNED PHYSICIAN OR SUPPLIER FOR SERVICE DESCRIBED BELOW

SIGNED (INSURED OR AUTHORIZED PERSON)

PHYSICIAN OR SUPPLIER INFORMATION

14. DATE OF: ◄ ILLNESS (FIRST SYMPTOM) OR INJURY (ACCIDENT) OR PREGNANCY (LMP)

15. DATE FIRST CONSULTED YOU FOR THIS CONDITION

16. IF PATIENT HAS HAD SAME OR SIMILAR ILLNESS OR INJURY, GIVE DATES

16.a. IF EMERGENCY CHECK HERE ☐

17. DATE PATIENT ABLE TO RETURN TO WORK

18. DATES OF TOTAL DISABILITY FROM THROUGH

DATES OF PARTIAL DISABILITY FROM THROUGH

19. NAME OF REFERRING PHYSICIAN OR OTHER SOURCE (e.g., PUBLIC HEALTH AGENCY)

20. FOR SERVICES RELATED TO HOSPITALIZATION GIVE HOSPITALIZATION DATES ADMITTED DISCHARGED

21. NAME & ADDRESS OF FACILITY WHERE SERVICES RENDERED (IF OTHER THAN HOME OR OFFICE)

22. WAS LABORATORY WORK PERFORMED OUTSIDE YOUR OFFICE? YES ☐ NO CHARGES

23. DIAGNOSIS OR NATURE OF ILLNESS OR INJURY. RELATE DIAGNOSIS TO PROCEDURE IN COLUMN D BY REFERENCE NUMBERS 1, 2, 3, ETC. OR DX CODE

1.
2.
3.
4.

B.
EPSDT YES ☐ NO ☐
FAMILY PLANNING YES ☐ NO ☐
PRIOR AUTHORIZATION NO.

24. DATE OF SERVICE FROM / TO	B* PLACE OF SERVICE	C FULLY DESCRIBE PROCEDURES, MEDICAL SERVICES OR SUPPLIES FURNISHED FOR EACH DATE GIVEN — PROCEDURE CODE (IDENTIFY:) / (EXPLAIN UNUSUAL SERVICES OR CIRCUMSTANCES)	D DIAGNOSIS CODE	E CHARGES	F DAYS OR UNITS	G* T.O.S.	H LEAVE BLANK

25. SIGNATURE OF PHYSICIAN OR SUPPLIER (INCLUDING DEGREE(S) OR CREDENTIALS) (I CERTIFY THAT THE STATEMENTS ON THE REVERSE APPLY TO THIS BILL AND ARE MADE A PART THEREOF)

26. ACCEPT ASSIGNMENT (GOVERNMENT CLAIMS ONLY) (SEE BACK) YES ☐ NO ☐

30. YOUR SOCIAL SECURITY NO.

27. TOTAL CHARGE

28. AMOUNT PAID

29. BALANCE DUE

31. PHYSICIAN'S SUPPLIERS AND OR GROUP NAME, ADDRESS, ZIP CODE AND TELEPHONE NO.

32. YOUR PATIENT'S ACCOUNT NO.

33. YOUR EMPLOYER ID NO.

ID NO.

*PLACE OF SERVICE AND TYPE OF SERVICE (T.O.S.) CODES ON BACK
REMARKS

APPROVED BY AMA COUNCIL ON MEDICAL SERVICE 6/83

FORM HCFA-1500 (1-84) FORM OWCP-1500
FORM CHAMPUS-501 (1-84) FORM RRB-1500

FORM AMA OP-503

HEALTH INSURANCE CLAIM FORM

(CHECK APPLICABLE PROGRAM BLOCK BELOW)

☐ MEDICARE (MEDICARE NO.) ☐ MEDICAID (MEDICAID NO.) ☐ CHAMPUS (SPONSOR'S SSN) ☐ CHAMPVA (VA FILE NO.) ☐ FECA BLACK LUNG (SSN) ☐ OTHER (CERTIFICATE SSN)

PATIENT AND INSURED (SUBSCRIBER) INFORMATION

PATIENT'S NAME (LAST NAME, FIRST NAME, MIDDLE INITIAL)	2. PATIENT'S DATE OF BIRTH	3. INSURED'S NAME (LAST NAME, FIRST NAME, MIDDLE INITIAL)
PATIENT'S ADDRESS (STREET, CITY, STATE, ZIP CODE)	5. PATIENT'S SEX MALE ☐ FEMALE ☐	6. INSURED'S ID NO. (FOR PROGRAM CHECKED ABOVE, INCLUDE ALL LETTERS)
	7. PATIENT'S RELATIONSHIP TO INSURED SELF ☐ SPOUSE ☐ CHILD ☐ OTHER ☐	8. INSURED'S GROUP NO. (OR GROUP NAME OR FECA CLAIM NO.) ☐ INSURED IS EMPLOYED AND COVERED BY EMPLOYER HEALTH PLAN
OTHER HEALTH INSURANCE COVERAGE (ENTER NAME OR POLICYHOLDER AND PLAN NAME AND ADDRESS AND POLICY OR MEDICAL ASSISTANCE NUMBER)	10. WAS CONDITION RELATED TO A. PATIENT'S EMPLOYMENT YES ☐ NO ☐ B. ACCIDENT AUTO ☐ OTHER ☐	11. INSURED'S ADDRESS (STREET, CITY, STATE, ZIP CODE) TELEPHONE NO. 11.a. CHAMPUS SPONSOR'S STATUS ☐ ACTIVE DUTY ☐ DECEASED BRANCH OF SERVICE ☐ RETIRED
PATIENT'S OR AUTHORIZED PERSON'S SIGNATURE (READ BACK BEFORE SIGNING) I AUTHORIZE THE RELEASE OF ANY MEDICAL INFORMATION NECESSARY TO PROCESS THIS CLAIM I ALSO REQUEST PAYMENT OF GOVERNMENT BENEFITS EITHER TO MYSELF OR TO THE PARTY WHO ACCEPTS ASSIGNMENT BELOW SIGNED DATE		13. I AUTHORIZE PAYMENT OF MEDICAL BENEFITS TO UNDERSIGNED PHYSICIAN OR SUPPLIER FOR SERVICE DESCRIBED BELOW SIGNED (INSURED OR AUTHORIZED PERSON)

PHYSICIAN OR SUPPLIER INFORMATION

DATE OF: ◀	ILLNESS (FIRST SYMPTOM) OR INJURY (ACCIDENT) OR PREGNANCY (LMP)	15. DATE FIRST CONSULTED YOU FOR THIS CONDITION	16. IF PATIENT HAS HAD SAME OR SIMILAR ILLNESS OR INJURY, GIVE DATES	16.a. IF EMERGENCY CHECK HERE ☐
DATE PATIENT ABLE TO RETURN TO WORK	18. DATES OF TOTAL DISABILITY FROM THROUGH		DATES OF PARTIAL DISABILITY FROM THROUGH	
NAME OF REFERRING PHYSICIAN OR OTHER SOURCE (e.g., PUBLIC HEALTH AGENCY)		20. FOR SERVICES RELATED TO HOSPITALIZATION GIVE HOSPITALIZATION DATES ADMITTED DISCHARGED	
NAME & ADDRESS OF FACILITY WHERE SERVICES RENDERED (IF OTHER THAN HOME OR OFFICE)		22. WAS LABORATORY WORK PERFORMED OUTSIDE YOUR OFFICE? YES ☐ NO ☐ CHARGES	

DIAGNOSIS OR NATURE OF ILLNESS OR INJURY. RELATE DIAGNOSIS TO PROCEDURE IN COLUMN D BY REFERENCE NUMBERS 1, 2, 3, ETC. OR DX CODE ──────┐

B.		
EPSDT	YES ☐	NO ☐
FAMILY PLANNING	YES ☐	NO ☐
PRIOR AUTHORIZATION NO.		

A DATE OF SERVICE FROM TO	B* PLACE OF SERVICE	C FULLY DESCRIBE PROCEDURES, MEDICAL SERVICES OR SUPPLIES FURNISHED FOR EACH DATE GIVEN PROCEDURE CODE (IDENTIFY:) (EXPLAIN UNUSUAL SERVICES OR CIRCUMSTANCES)	D DIAGNOSIS CODE	E CHARGES	F DAYS OR UNITS	G* T.O.S.	H LEAVE BLANK

SIGNATURE OF PHYSICIAN OR SUPPLIER (INCLUDING DEGREE(S) OR CREDENTIALS) (I CERTIFY THAT THE STATEMENTS ON THE REVERSE APPLY TO THIS BILL AND ARE MADE A PART THEREOF)	26. ACCEPT ASSIGNMENT (GOVERNMENT CLAIMS ONLY) (SEE BACK) YES ☐ NO ☐	27. TOTAL CHARGE	28. AMOUNT PAID	29. BALANCE DUE
	30. YOUR SOCIAL SECURITY NO.	31. PHYSICIAN'S SUPPLIERS AND OR GROUP NAME, ADDRESS, ZIP CODE AND TELEPHONE NO.		
YOUR PATIENT'S ACCOUNT NO.	33. YOUR EMPLOYER ID NO.	ID NO.		

PLACE OF SERVICE AND TYPE OF SERVICE (T.O.S.) CODES ON BACK   REMARKS

APPROVED BY AMA COUNCIL ON MEDICAL SERVICE 6/83

FORM HCFA-1500 (1-84) FORM OWCP-1500
FORM CHAMPUS-501 (1-84) FORM RRB-1500

FORM AMA OP-503

PATIENT'S REQUEST FOR MEDICARE PAYMENT

IMPORTANT— SEE OTHER SIDE FOR INSTRUCTIONS

PLEASE TYPE OR PRINT INFORMATION

MEDICAL INSURANCE BENEFITS SOCIAL SECURITY ACT

NOTICE: Anyone who misrepresents or falsifies essential information requested by this form may upon conviction be subject to fine and imprisonment under Federal Law. No Part B Medicare benefits may be paid unless this form is received as required by existing law and regulations (20 CFR 422.510).

1 Name of Beneficiary From Health Insurance Card

(First)   (Middle)   (Last)

SEND COMPLETED FORM TO:

MEDICARE
PENNSYLVANIA BLUE SHIELD
BOX 65
CAMP HILL, PA. 17011

2 Claim Number From Health Insurance Card

☐ Male
☐ Female

3 Patient's Mailing Address (City, State, Zip Code)
Check here if this is a new address ➡ ☐

(Street or P.O. Box—Include Apartment number)

(City)   (State)   (Zip)

3b Telephone Number
(Include Area Code)

4 Describe The Illness or Injury for Which Patient Received Treatment

4b Was illness or injury connected with employment?

☐ Yes
☐ No

If any medical expenses will be or could be paid by your private insurance organization, State Agency, (Medicaid), or the VA complete block 5 below.

5 Name and Address of other insurance, State Agency (Medicaid), or VA office

Policy or Medical
Assistance Number

NOTE: If you DO NOT want payment information on this claim released put an (x) here ➡ ☐

I authorize Any Holder of Medical or Other Information About Me to Release to the Social Security Administration and Health Care Financing Administration or Its Intermediaries or Carriers any Information Needed for This or a Related Medicare Claim. I Permit copy of this Authorization to be Used in Place of the Original, and Request Payment of Medical Insurance Benefits to Me.

6 Signature of Patient (If patient is unable to sign, see Block 6 on other side.)

6b Date Signed

IMPORTANT!

ATTACH ITEMIZED BILLS FROM YOUR DOCTOR(S)
OR SUPPLIER(S) TO THE BACK OF THIS FORM.

HCFA-1490S (6-80)

Department of Health and Human Services—Health Care Financing Administration

CHAPTER 14

INSURANCE FOR THE
DOCTOR AND STAFF

QUIZ

A. From the items listed under each question, select the correct answer or answers. Write the corresponding letter or letters in the answer space.

1. A doctor's workers' compensation insurance would cover:
   a. injury to a serviceman while repairing equipment in the office.
   b. salaries paid to employees while on temporary layoff.
   c. salaries paid to the medical assistant unable to work because of illness.
   d. medical expenses of employees injured while working.   _____

2. A doctor might bond his medical assistant in order to:
   a. insure against loss if the assistant took office funds for personal use.
   b. provide supplemental income for the assistant.
   c. insure against theft of cash from the assistant while enroute to the bank.
   d. insure against loss of cash as a result of burglary of the office.   _____

3. When a doctor owns the building in which his or her office is located, insurance should include coverage for:
   a. fire, smoke, lightning, windstorm and other causes of damage to the building.
   b. liability for injury to someone falling on a poorly maintained inside stairway.
   c. liability for injury to someone who slips on the front walk leading to the building.
   d. liability for injury to a patient while parking in an adjoining public parking lot.   _____

4. Which of the following wrongful actions by a medical assistant would be covered by the assistant's malpractice insurance?
   a. Overcharging patients who pay cash and keeping the extra amounts.
   b. Revealing patient's health problems outside the office.
   c. Inadvertently using an unsterile hypodermic needle.
   d. Leading a patient to believe the doctor could cure an ailment.   _____

5. In the case of a fire insurance policy based on current value of the insured property, which of the following would be useful in making a claim?
   a. Photographs of the office.
   b. Original invoices for the equipment at time of purchase.
   c. Purchase dates of furnishings.
   d. Cost of replacing damaged property with new.
   _____

6. In the case of a doctor, insurance against "income loss" would generally cover which of the following situations?
   a. Heart attack which kept the doctor out of the office for six weeks.
   b. A winter storm which caused the office to shut down for two days.
   c. Long term disabling injury to a partner in the doctor's group practice.
   d. Long term illness of the medical assistant.
   _____

The following two questions relate to situations in which the medical assistant's handling can minimize the risk of professional liability claims against the doctor.

7. You are about to draw a blood sample and the patient questions the necessity of the procedure. Would you:
   a. assure the patient that there will be no pain?
   b. stop and recheck with the doctor before proceeding?
   c. explain that such testing is routine with all patients?
   d. tell the patient the test is necessary because the doctor has ordered it?
   _____

8. You overhear a patient remark that the doctor's treatment seems to be aggravating the problem rather than relieving it. The patient has a history of complaining and being difficult to work with. Would you:
   a. at the first opportunity tell the doctor what the patient said?
   b. avoid carrying tales?
   c. assure the patient that the experiences of others with similar ailments are about the same?
   d. suggest to the doctor that the patient's bill might be reduced?
   _____

B. 1. List six categories of insurance that a doctor with an office practice would probably carry for his own protection.

   1. _____   4. _____

   2. _____   5. _____

   3. _____   6. _____

2. List five causes of damage or loss that would probably be covered by a doctor's insurance on office property.

   1. _____   4. _____

   2. _____   5. _____

   3. _____

3. List five items of property which a doctor's fire insurance should be designed to cover in a rented office.

   1. _____   4. _____

   2. _____   5. _____

   3. _____   _____

4. Name two good places for the safekeeping of an inventory of office property.

   1. _____

   2. _____

      _____

5. You are making the annual review of office property to determine whether to increase the amount of fire-insurance coverage on a policy based on replacement values. Name three types of changes you would consider.

   1. _____

   2. _____

   3. _____

ACTICE AND PROJECTS

Your doctor-employer is seriously injured in an automobile accident, is unreachable in intensive care for a week, and is not expected to return to practice for six months. What types of insurance policies would you look for among the doctor's papers and what losses or expenses might such insurance policies cover? Limit your answer to about 50 words or less.

_____

_____

_____

_____

_____

_____

_____

_____

_____

B. You are taking an electrocardiogram and the machine stops operating. Briefly explain how you would react and what you would tell the patient. Limit your answer to about 50 words.

_____

_____

_____

_____

_____

_____

C. Look up the basic provisions of the current physicians' malpractice legislation in your state and write a brief summary of the limitations or other procedures which have been set up to restrain the rising cost of malpractice claims. Possible sources of this information are the local library, the County Medical Society, or your representative in the State Legislature. Write about 50 words or less.

_____

_____

_____

_____

_____

D. Select a classroom or section of the school laboratory and make an inventory of the contents which would be used to support a fire insurance claim. To the extent possible, list manufacturer's name and model numbers for major items. Estimate date of purchase and purchase price.

_____

_____

_____

_____

_____

_____

_____

_____

CHAPTER 15

PROTECTION THROUGH STERILIZATION AND DISINFECTION

In the blank spaces provided, write the answers to the following questions.

1. What is the name given to the study of fungi? _____

2. What is the name given to the study of viruses? _____

3. What method of killing bacteria will insure the destruction of spores?

   _____

4. On what principle does an autoclave operate? _____

5. Which form of microorganism causes the following diseases?

   a. Athlete's foot _____

   b. Rocky Mountain spotted fever _____

   c. Malaria _____

   d. Strep throat _____

   e. Syphillis _____

   f. Tuberculosis _____

   g. Measles _____

6. Which is lighter—steam or air? _____

7. Which will more rapidly penetrate a package wrapped in porous covering for

   sterilization—steam or hot air? _____

8. a. What is the typical temperature for autoclaving? _____

   b. How long is this temperature usually sustained
   for metal and glass items? _____

9. a. Which method of sterilizing requires higher
        temperature—autoclaving or dry heat?_____

    b. Which method requires more time?_____

10. A package of disposable surgical gloves is opened but not used. Should the
    gloves be kept in the package until the next scheduled surgery or discarded?

    _____

B. From the words, phrases, or statements following each question, select the one o
    ones that correctly answer the question. Write the corresponding letter or
    letters in the answer space.

    1. Which of the following are microorganisms?
        a. Viruses
        b. Vectors
        c. Fungi
        d. Staphylococci
        e. Microns
        f. Microscopic algae
        g. Amebas   _____

    2. Viruses are able to exist only in what type of environment?
        a. Outside the human organism
        b. Inside the human organism
        c. Within the living cells of other organisms
        d. In ambiant temperatures
        e. In diseased tissues   _____

    3. Which of the following are chemical disinfectants?
        a. Formaldehyde
        b. Lysol
        c. 70 to 90% isopropyl alcohol
        d. Sodium chloride
        e. Precipitated calcium carbonate   _____

    4. In wrapping packs for autoclaving, which of the following
        represent(s) correct practice?
        a. An individual pack should include only items that are
            expected to be used at one time.
        b. Items to be sterilized should be completely covered by
            the wrapping.
        c. The wrapping should be tight and firm.
        d. Sterilization indicators should be securely attached
            to the exterior of each pack.
        e. Syringes should be disassembled.   _____

    5. Which is the principal reason for using disposable equipment
        in a doctor's office?
        a. It virtually eliminates the danger of inadequate sterilization.
        b. It is more economical than reuseable equipment.
        c. It reflects more modern office practice.
        d. It eliminates the time-consuming process of sterilization. _____

6. Eucaryotic microorganisms have which of the following characteristics?
   a. Multiple cell structure
   b. More than one chromosome in a cell
   c. Membranes separating various functioning structures within a cell
   d. Reproduction by binary fission   _____

7. Procaryotic organisms are:
   a. structurally more primitive than eucaryotic organisms.
   b. able to reproduce by the process of mitosis.
   c. without distinguishable organ structures.
   d. larger than viruses.   _____

8. Which of the following are proper procedures for sanitizing
   used instruments?
   a. Place them in boiling water.
   b. Polish bright metal surfaces.
   c. Use gloves if you have breaks in the skin of your hands.
   d. Soak instruments in detergent until they can be more
      thoroughly scrubbed.   _____

9. Which of the following procedures should be followed in
   disinfecting instruments with boiling water?
   a. Instruments need not be submerged in the water.
   b. Boiling time should be about 20-30 minutes.
   c. Distilled water should be used.
   d. Instruments should be wrapped before placing them
      in the boiling unit.   _____

10. Which of the following are proper procedures to be followed in
    wrapping a set of two instruments in porous paper for autoclaving?
    a. Instruments should not be touching.
    b. A corner of the package may be left open to permit
       identification of contents after autoclaving.
    c. Wrap must be folded so that when the package is opened the
       wrapping can be unfolded without touching the instruments.
    d. A tape used to keep the wrapping closed should be marked
       to identify contents and show date of autoclaving.   _____

1. List below four forms of microscopic life.

   1. _____   3. _____

   2. _____   4. _____

2. List below the three major morphological groups of bacteria and indicate
   their general shapes.

   1. _____

   2. _____

   3. _____

3. List below two units of measurement used currently for microorganisms, giving the symbols and fractional part of a meter for each.

    1. _____

    2. _____

4. Name three methods of sterilization.

    1. _____

    2. _____

    3. _____

5. Name three methods of disinfection.

    1. _____

    2. _____

    3. _____

6. Name three conditions which may be measured by sterilization indicators.

    1. _____

    2. _____

    3. _____

7. List five characteristics common to all living organisms.

    1. _____

    2. _____

    3. _____

    4. _____

    5. _____

D. 1. Read the following definitions pertaining to control of microorganisms. For each definition select from the column at the right the term that best matches it. Write the term in the answer space in the center.

DEFINITION	ANSWER	TERM
(1) Material capable of preventing growth or action of microorganisms without necessarily killing them.	(1)_____	a. Disinfection
(2) Process of destroying most microorganisms but usually not spores.	(2)_____	b. Stasis
(3) Condition of arrested growth.	(3)_____	c. Antiseptic
(4) Free from disease-producing microorganisms.	(4)_____	d. Sterile
(5) Free of all living microorganisms.	(5)_____	e. Aseptic
(6) Capable of causing a disease.	(6)_____	f. Germicide
(7) Affected by disease-producing microorganisms.	(7)_____	g. Contaminated
(8) Material capable of killing germs.	(8)_____	h. Pathogenic
(9) Material capable of killing fungi.	(9)_____	i. Septic
(10) Infected or made impure by contact with unsterile objects.	(10)_____	j. Fungicide
(11) Process of destroying all microorganisms including spores.	(11)_____	k. Sterilization

2. Read the following definitions pertaining to microbiology. For each definition select from the column at the right the term that best matches it. Write the term in the answer space in the center.

DEFINITION	ANSWER	TERM
(1) Constructed first lens strong enough to detect microorganisms.	(1)_____	a. Robert Koch
(2) Known as father of bacteriology.	(2)_____	b. Bacilli
(3) Originated modern antiseptic technique.	(3)_____	c. Amorphous
(4) Isolated tubercle bacillus.	(4)_____	d. Eucaryote
(5) Cell having a true nucleus.	(5)_____	e. Protozoa
(6) The study and science of bacteria.	(6)_____	f. Streptococci
(7) An agent that carries infecting microorganisms.	(7)_____	g. Anton van Leeuwenhoek
(8) Single-celled, non-parasitic eucaryote.	(8)_____	h. Staphylococci

(9) Splitting in two.	(9)_____	i. Spirilla
(10) Spiral-shaped bacteria.	(10)_____	j. Lister
(11) Pertaining to shape, appearance.	(11)_____	k. Bacteriology
(12) Spherical bacteria.	(12)_____	l. Diplococci
(13) Rod-shaped bacteria.	(13)_____	m. Morphologic
(14) Grapelike clusters of cocci.	(14)_____	n. Pasteur
(15) Forming pairs of cells.	(15)_____	o. Vector
(16) Forming chains of cells.	(16)_____	p. Cocci
(17) Not having definite shape.	(17)_____	q. Binary fission
(18) Relative degree of infectiousness of a microorganism.	(18)_____	r. Virus
(19) A mold or mushroom.	(19)_____	s. Fungus
(20) Ultramicroscopic parasite.	(20)_____	t. Virulence

PRACTICE AND PROJECTS

A. A pair of forceps has been used in treating a patient. Describe the detailed steps that should be followed in sterilizing the instrument by autoclave for storage.

_____

_____

_____

_____

_____

_____

_____

_____

_____

B. 1. Explain briefly why sterilization indicators should be used.

_____

_____

_____

2. Explain where sterilization indicators are placed and why.

_____

_____

3. State why some sterilization indicators have long ends or have strings attached to them.

_____

_____

4. From the following drawings identify each morphologic group of bacteria. Using Figures 15-3, 15-4, and 15-5 in the text, write in the identity of each form of bacteria below each group.

a. _____   b. _____   c. _____

15-3   15-4   15-5

A. _____   A. _____   A. _____

B. _____   B. _____   B. _____

C. _____   C. _____   C. _____

D. _____   D. _____   D. _____

E. _____   E. _____

                       F. _____

                       G. _____

                       H. _____

                       I. _____

115

CHAPTER 16

ASSISTING WITH EXAMINATIONS

Complete the following statements:

1. The medical term for an abnormally fast pulse is _____.

2. The medical term for an abnormally slow pulse is _____.

3. An average pulse rate for most healthy persons would be in the range of _____ to _____ per minute.

4. The thumb should not be used to feel a patient's pulse, because it has its own _____.

5. Children's pulse rates are frequently _____ than adults.

6. The normal number of breaths per minute is about _____ to _____.

7. The normal number of pulse beats per breath is about _____.

8. A respiration consists of one _____ and one _____.

9. Exhaled air contains a larger proportion of _____ and a smaller proportion of _____.

10. Shallow breathing results in insufficient _____.

11. Labored breathing is referred to as _____.

12. Normal vision is recorded as _____.

13. An instrument for opening and holding open an entrance into the interior of the body is called a _____.

14. Loss of body heat is slowed when blood vessels _____.

15. Perspiration is the body's way of _____ temperature.

16. Normal oral temperature is _____ Fahrenheit and _____ Celsiu

17. Normal rectal temperature is _____ Fahrenheit and _____ Celsiu

18. Axillary temperatures are taken in the _____ and are _____ than oral temperatures.

19. A mercury thermometer should always be rinsed in _____ water.

20. The force at which the blood surges through the arterial system is called

_____.

B. From the items below each question, select the one that is the correct answer. Write the corresponding letter in the answer space.

1. Which of the following would best describe examination by means of palpatio
   a. Touching
   b. Feeling or manipulation with the hands
   c. Sensing of palpitations
   d. Squeezing   _____

2. What is an average blood-pressure reading for persons under 40 years of age?
   a. 75/125   c. 100/60
   b. 120/80   d. 150/75   _____

3. What general principle should be followed in draping a patient?
   a. Leave uncovered those areas the doctor will be examining.
   b. Use disposable sheeting as much as possible.
   c. Allow the patient to adjust the covering to his or her own choice.
   d. The patient should not be exposed until the doctor is ready to examine.   _____

4. An oral temperature reading may not be valid when it is affected by which of the following factors?
   a. Exercise   c. Elevated blood pressure
   b. Rapid breathing   d. Fever   _____

5. Before taking an oral temperature, the assistant should check to see that the thermometer does not read higher than what level?
   a. 98.6°F
   b. 96.0°F
   c. 37.0°C
   d. The lowest degree marked on the thermometer   _____

6. Which of the following examination procedures would be classified as auscultation?
   a. Using a stethoscope to hear beartbeats
   b. Taking a pulse
   c. Feeling for fetal heartbeats
   d. Observing the reaction of pupils to light.   _____

7. Which of the following is a correct statement in regard to
   measuring the visual acuity of a patient?
   a. 20/80 vision indicates the patient is farsighted.
   b. 20/10 vision indicates the patient is farsighted.
   c. 20/80 is a valid measurement of near vision.
   d. 40/20 is a valid measurement of visual acuity.   _____

1. Name six methods used in physical examinations.

   1. _____   4. _____

   2. _____   5. _____

   3. _____   6. _____

2. Name six parts of an examination that may often be performed by the medical
   assistant.

   1. _____   4. _____

   2. _____   5. _____

   3. _____   6. _____

3. List at least five things the medical assistant should do in preparing the
   patient for examination.

   1. _____

   2. _____

   3. _____

   4. _____

   5. _____

   _____

   _____

4. Name at least four physical factors on which blood pressure depends.

   1. _____

   2. _____

   3. _____

   4. _____

   _____

5. Name two other factors that may influence blood pressure.

1. _____   2. _____

6. What are the four "vital signs"?

1. _____   3. _____

2. _____   4. _____

7. Rank the three methods of taking temperatures in descending order of accuracy.

Most accurate: _____

Fairly accurate: _____

Least accurate: _____

8. To judge the adequacy of blood flow to various parts of the body, the docto may feel the pulse at various locations. Name three of these locations.

1. _____

2. _____

3. _____

_____

_____

9. You are directed to prepare a male patient for an abdominal examination. What instructions would you give to the patient so that he would be ready for the doctor to proceed with the examination?

_____

_____

_____

_____

_____

10. Describe two ways in which you might drape a patient in the lithotomy position using a plain rectangular sheet.

1. _____

2. _____

_____

Read the definitions given below. For each definition, select from the column to the right the term that best matches it. Write the term in the answer space in the center.

DEFINITION	ANSWER	TERM
1. Period when the heart contracts forcing blood into the arteries.	1. _____	a. Pulse pressure
2. Instrument for examining the inner eye.	2. _____	b. Systole
3. Minimum pressure when heart is relaxed.	3. _____	c. Diastole
4. Below normal blood pressure.	4. _____	d. Hypertension
5. Maximum pressure exerted by heartbeat.	5. _____	e. Hypotension
6. Period when the heart rests and arteries are returning to normal size.	6. _____	f. Sphygmomanometer
7. Instrument for measuring blood pressure.	7. _____	g. Systolic pressure
8. Instrument for listening to sounds made within the body.	8. _____	h. Diastolic pressure
9. Above normal blood pressure.	9. _____	i. Unit for measuring blood pressure
10. mmHg (millimeters of mercury).	10. _____	j. Ophthalmoscope
11. Instrument for inspecting the ear.	11. _____	k. Otoscope
12. Difference between systolic and diastolic pressure.	12. _____	l. Speculum
13. Instrument for opening an entrance to the body.	13. _____	m. Stethoscope
14. Lettering used to assess distant vision.	14. _____	n. Sigmoidoscope
15. Instrument for examining the rectum.	15. _____	o. Snellen chart

PRACTICE AND PROJECTS

A. Name the instruments pictured below and the purpose for which they are used.

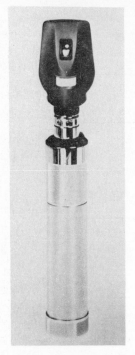

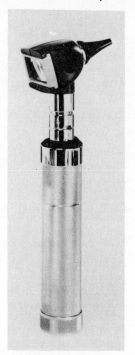

1. _____

2. _____

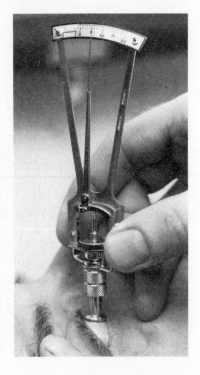

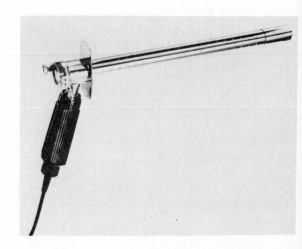

3. _____

4. _____

8. Name the positions for examining patients according to the numbered pictures below.

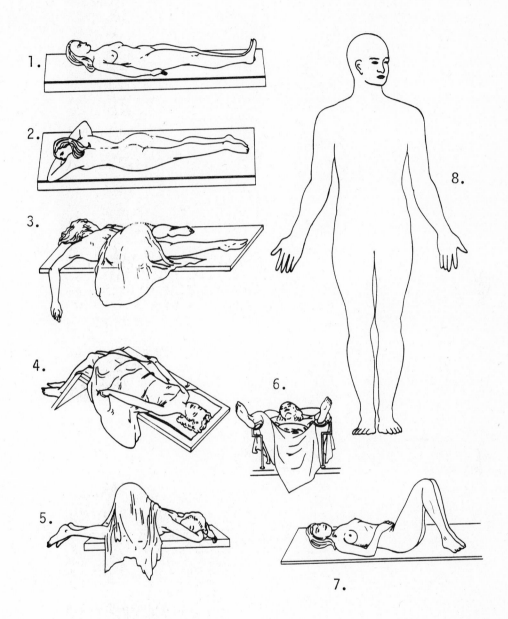

1. _____

2. _____

3. _____

4. _____

5. _____

6. _____

7. _____

8. _____

CHAPTER 17

THE OFFICE LABORATORY

. Complete the following statements relating to the microscope.

1. An ocular marked 10X means a magnification of _____.

2. To achieve a magnification of 1000 _____ with a microscope having 10X oculars, an objective of _____ must be used.

3. Immersion oil has the same _____ power as glass, and therefore when using the oil-immersion objective a minimum of _____ is lost.

4. In order to move a slide smoothly and precisely, a _____ stage is used.

5. The condenser serves to _____ light on the object under study.

6. The _____ power objective is used for initial positioning and focusing of the slide.

7. Objects in the _____ of a field of vision will provide the best view.

8. A microscope with two oculars is described as _____.

9. When using the oil-immersion objective, _____ light is needed than for the other objectives.

10. The opening of the iris diaphragm can be made _____ in order to allow more _____ to be directed at the object.

. From the items below each question, select the correct answer or answers. Write the corresponding letter or letters in the answer space.

1. If the pH of a urine specimen were 8, it would be which of the following?
   a. Acid   c. Neutral
   b. Alkaline   d. Amphoteric   _____

2. Which of the following is the normal range of specific gravity of urine?
   a. 1.002 to 1.010   c. 1.010 to 1.025
   b. 1.005 to 1.015   d. 1.015 to 1.030   _____

3. In an RBC pipet, if blood is taken to the 0.5 mark and diluted to the 101 mark, what will be the dilution?
   a. 1:50
   b. 1:100
   c. 1:150
   d. 1:200

4. In counting RBCs, what is the correct number of squares in which cells must be counted?
   a. 5 squares
   b. 4 squares
   c. 3 squares
   d. 2 squares

5. Which of the following is a polymorphonuclear cell?
   a. Lymphocyte
   b. Platelet
   c. Eosinophil
   d. Erythrocyte

6. What is a distinguishing characteristic of the nucleus in a polymorphonuclear cell?
   a. It is round and stains deep purple.
   b. It is kidney-shaped.
   c. It has several lobes with connecting strands of chromatin.
   d. All the above

7. In a WBC pipet, if the blood is drawn to the 0.5 mark and diluted to the 11 mark, what is the resulting dilution?
   a. 1:5
   b. 1:10
   c. 1:20
   d. 1:30

8. In reporting results of examining a bacteriological smear, the medical assistant should:
   a. identify bacteria as to genus and species.
   b. describe shape and grouping.
   c. describe staining reaction.
   d. count individual cells.

9. What is the minimum number of cells to count when examining a differential smear?
   a. 50
   b. 100
   c. 150
   d. 200

10. When examining a bacteriological smear under the microscope, which is the proper objective to use?
    a. Oil immersion
    b. Low power
    c. High power
    d. Any of the above

11. Which of the following statements are procedures to follow in caring for a microscope?
    a. The microscope should be covered when the office is closed.
    b. Paper towels may be used to brush dust from lenses.
    c. A special "lens paper" should be used to wipe lenses.
    d. Make certain your fingers are washed thoroughly before touching the lenses.

12. Which of the following are proper procedures in preparing a bacteriological smear?
    a. The swab holding the material to be examined should be rolled over the slide.
    b. The swab holding the material to be examined should be wiped over the slide lightly.
    c. Heat may be used to dry the smear more quickly.
    d. Fixing the smear requires brief flaming on the side of the slide that does not have the smear on it.

    _____

1. Name the five types of white cells reported in a differential count.

    1. _____ 4. _____

    2. _____ 5. _____

    3. _____

2. List five types of tissue which should not be used as a site for skin puncture.

    1. _____ 4. _____

    2. _____ 5. _____

    3. _____

3. Name three types of casts found in urine.

    1. _____ 2. _____ 3. _____

4. List four sites that can be used for a skin puncture: two most common for adults and two for infants.

    1. _____

    2. _____

    3. _____

    4. _____

5. List the five tests included in a complete blood count.

    1. _____ 4. _____

    2. _____ 5. _____

    3. _____

6. List the usual tests performed in a routine urinalysis.

    1. _____ 4. _____ 6. _____

    2. _____ 5. _____ 7. _____

    3. _____   _____

7. The following are some steps to take to adjust a microscope to examine a slide under high power. Indicate the order in which you would take these steps by placing a number in the space for each step.

    ____ Raise the objective and clamp the slide on the stage.

    ____ Move the slide so that the object is directly in the center of the field of vision.

    ____ Swing the high power objective into viewing position and focus with the fine adjustment.

    ____ Set the low power objective close to the slide, raise with the coarse adjustment until in the approximate focus.

    ____ Use the fine adjustment to get the best low power focus.

8. Name four constituents of urine other than glucose and protein that often are part of the chemical analysis of urine.

    1. _____   3. _____

    2. _____   4. _____

9. Indicate what would be normal for each of the following characteristics of urine.

    1. pH   _____

    2. Specific gravity _____

    3. Casts   _____

10. Name three results that can be interpreted from culture studies of urine.

    1. _____

    2. _____

    3. _____

11. Name the three formed elements of blood.

    1. _____ 2. _____ 3. _____

12. Indicate the order in which the following steps would be taken in the Gram stain technique.

    ____ Apply 95% ethyl alcohol to smear and allow to run off three times; rinse with water.

    ____ Cover smear with Gram's iodine; rinse with water.

    ____ Cover smear with gentian violet; rinse with water.

    ____ Apply safranine or dilute fuchsin; rinse with water.

128

13. The steps in question C-12 may be described in one or two words. Indicate which of the above steps goes with the following words.

_____ Fix   _____ Primary stain

_____ Counterstain   _____ Decolorize

Read the definitions given below. For each definition select from the column at the right the term that best matches it. Write the term in the answer space in the center.

DEFINITION	ANSWER	TERM
1. Classification of WBCs	1. _____	a. Ocular
2. Retain deep purple stain	2. _____	b. Oil immersion
3. Weight relative to that of distilled water	3. _____	c. pH
4. Eyepiece	4. _____	d. Specific gravity
5. Bacteria stained red or pink.	5. _____	e. Erythrocyte
6. Used for blood-cell identification	6. _____	f. Leukocyte
7. Highest-power objective	7. _____	g. Hypochromia
8. White blood cell	8. _____	h. Differential
9. Denotes acidity or alkalinity	9. _____	i. Hematocrit
10. Red blood cell	10. _____	j. Platelets
11. Hemoglobin test measurement	11. _____	k. Gram-positive bacteria
12. Having multilobed nuclei	12. _____	l. 10,000
13. Clot cells	13. _____	m. Polymorphonuclear cells
14. Increased pallor in red cells	14. _____	n. Grams/100 milliliters
15. Percent volume of packed RBCs after centrifugation	15. _____	o. Wright's stain
16. Top fluid after centrifuging urine	16. _____	p. Cuvette
17. Multiplier used in making white blood cell count	17. _____	q. Supernatant
18. Glass tube for holding specimen in colorimeter	18. _____	r. mm^3

19. Microliter   19. _____   s. 50

20. Multiplier used in making   20. _____   t. Gram-negative
    red blood cell count   bacteria

PRACTICE AND PROJECTS

A. Explain in your own words why the tissue around the puncture site on a finger
   should not be squeezed hard when blood is being taken.

   _____

   _____

B. Briefly outline in your own words the steps you would take in obtaining blood by
   venipuncture, with the Vacutainer system.

   _____

   _____

   _____

   _____

   _____

   _____

   _____

   _____

   _____

   _____

   _____

   _____

   _____

   _____

   _____

   _____

_____

_____

_____

_____

_____

_____

In the picture below, count the leukocytes and place the number in the blank space provided. What power would you use on the microscope?

_____ leukocytes in 1 mm^2

_____ power used

Fill in the approximate normals for the following blood tests.

TEST	NORMAL - -MAN	NORMAL - -WOMAN
1. Hemoglobin		
2. Hematocrit		
3. Red-blood cell count		
4. White-blood cell count		
5. Neutrophils		
6. Lymphocytes		
7. Monocytes		
8. Eosinophils		
9. Basophils		
10. Erythrocyte sedimentation rate (Wintrobe method)		

E. List instructions you would give to a female patient for obtaining a clean, mid-stream catch urine specimen.

_____

_____

_____

_____

_____

_____

_____

_____

CHAPTER 18

ELECTROCARDIOGRAPHY AND PULMONARY FUNCTION

QUIZ

A. Complete the following statements:

1. The heart goes through its pumping cycle about _____ times a day.

2. Oxygenated blood is carried from the _____ to the _____ in the pulmonary veins.

3. The pulmonary artery carries deoxygenated blood from the _____ to the _____.

4. The sinoatrial node is also called the _____.

5. The common practice in taking an electrocardiogram is to make a tracing of each of _____ lead circuits.

6. It is usually easier to have the electrocardiograph on the _____ side of the patient.

7. The ground electrode for an electrocardiograph is attached to the _____ _____.

8. On electrocardiograph paper the vertical scale measures _____ and the horizontal scale measures _____.

9. The front side of electrocardiograph paper is sensitive to _____.

10. When an ECG tracing is to be rolled into a coil, start the coil with the _____ lead and finish with lead _____ in the outside wrap.

11. In ventilation testing, all breathing is through the _____.

B. From the items below each question, select the correct answer or answers. Write the corresponding letter or letters in the answer space.

1. The correct standardization deflection on electrocardiograph paper is:
   a. five 1-mm divisions.
   b. eight 1-mm divisions.
   c. ten 1-mm divisions.
   d. fifteen 1-mm divisions.   _____

2. Electrical impulses measured in electrocardiography are those produced by the:
   a. electrocardiograph.
   c. patient's own body.
   b. electrodes.
   d. lead circuits.

   _____

3. Electrocardiograph paper normally moves at a speed of:
   a. 50 mm per second.
   c. 10 mm per second.
   b. 5 inches per second.
   d. 25 mm per second.

   _____

4. On electrocardiograph paper one millivolt equals:
   a. one light line on the vertical scale.
   b. two heavy lines on the horizontal scale.
   c. two heavy lines on the vertical scale.
   d. one heavy line on the vertical scale.

   _____

5. On electrocardiograph paper one second equals:
   a. one heavy line on the vertical scale.
   b. one heavy line on the horizontal scale.
   c. five heavy lines on the horizontal scale.
   d. five heavy lines on the vertical scale.

   _____

6. Which of the following might affect the accuracy of an electrocardiogram?
   a. Patient's temperature above normal.
   b. Nearby electrical appliances and/or equipment.
   c. Restlessless of patient during test.
   d. Patient in contact with metal examination table.
   e. Patient with artificial lower right leg.

   _____

7. Which of the following represent good practice in placement of ECG electrodes?
   a. Straps holding limb electrodes should be pulled as tight as possible to get best conduction.
   b. Electrodes may be attached on any fleshy part of the arms.
   c. Electrode jelly should be spread across the chest before chest electrodes are applied.
   d. Reuseable electrodes should be cleaned with alcohol after each use.

   _____

8. Which of the following represent good practice in mounting ECG tracings?
   a. Cut up and mount only one patient's tracing at a time.
   b. Note any nonstandard speed for the tracing.
   c. Exclude any abnormal complexes when trimming a tracing.
   d. Be sure each position of the tracing for mounting includes identification of the lead.

   _____

C. 1. Indicate where you would place the electrode in each of the following chest leads:

   V1. _____

   V2. _____

   V3. _____

V4. _____

_____

V5. _____

V6. _____

_____

2. Name three common types of measurements of ventilation. Also show the abbreviation for each.

1. _____

2. _____

3. _____

3. Various parts of the heart and connecting blood vessels are listed below. In the blank spaces on the right, rearrange these parts and vessels in the order in which blood passes through them.

Right atrium   1. _____

Left atrium   2. _____

Right ventricle   3. _____

Left ventricle   4. _____

Aorta   5. _____

Pulmonary artery   6. _____

Pulmonary vein   7. _____

Tricuspid valve   8. _____

Mitral valve   9. _____

4. The parts of the heart that initiate and transmit impulses to the heart muscles are listed below. In the blank spaces on the right, rearrange these parts in the order in which the impulses flow during a pumping cycle.

Atrioventricular node   1. _____

Bundle of His   2. _____

Purkinje fibers   3. _____

Sinoatrial node   4. _____

5. a. For the 12 leads listed below write in the code markings in dots (...)
      and dashes (---).

   b. From the circuits listed directly below, select the proper one for each
      of the first six leads and write it in the space provided.

CIRCUITS

Right arm—combination left leg and left arm
Right arm—left leg
Right arm—left arm
Left arm —combination left leg and right arm
Left arm —left leg
Left leg —combination right and left arms

CODE		CIRCUIT
1. Lead 1	_____	_____
2. Lead 2	_____	_____
3. Lead 3	_____	_____
4. Lead aVR	_____	_____
5. Lead aVL	_____	_____
6. Lead aVF	_____	_____
7. Lead V1	_____	
8. Lead V2	_____	
9. Lead V3	_____	
10. Lead V4	_____	
11. Lead V5	_____	
12. Lead V6	_____	

6. Name the two kinds of capacity that make up the total air capacity of the
   lungs.

   1. _____   2. _____

D. For each definition below, select the term that best matches it from the column
   at the right. Write the term you select in the answer column.

DEFINITION	ANSWER	TERM
1. Device to record electrical heart action.	1. _____	a. artifacts
2. Device to record volume of air exhaled.	2. _____	b. echocardiography

3.	Device to measure physical effort	3._____	c.	electrocardiogram
4.	Writing arm on electro-cardiograph	4._____	d.	electrocardiograph
5.	Graphic tracing of electrical heart action	5._____	e.	ergometer
6.	Contraction of atria	6._____	f.	P wave
7.	Contraction of ventricles	7._____	g.	QRS wave
8.	Recovery (repolarization) of ventricles	8._____	h.	T wave
9.	Erroneous movements of ECG stylus	9._____	i.	spirometer
10.	Use of ultrasound to show heart structure and movement	10._____	j.	stylus

PRACTICE AND PROJECTS

A. State in your own words how you would check to determine if an electrocardio-graph were standardized.

_____

_____

_____

B. On the sample electrocardiograph paper pictured below, draw a typical electro-cardiogram tracing of one complete heart beat, labeling the P, Q, R, S, and T points. Also draw a correct standardization deflection.

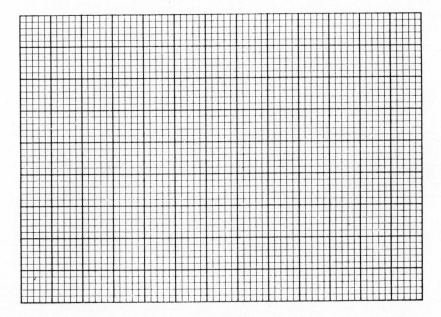

C. List the steps you would take to prepare a patient for an electrocardiogram.

_____

_____

_____

_____

_____

_____

D. You are about to give a patient three ventilation tests:

   a. How would you explain each test to the patient?
   b. What instructions would you give the patient about each test?
   c. What general breathing instructions apply to all these tests?

    1. Vital capacity

      a. _____

         _____

      b. _____

         _____

    2. Forced expiratory volume

      a. _____

         _____

      b. _____

         _____

    3. Maximum voluntary ventilation

      a. _____

         _____

      b. _____

         _____

   c. General breathing instructions applying to all tests:

      _____

      _____

CHAPTER 19

X-RAYS AND RELATED PROCEDURES— PRINCIPLES AND PATIENT PREPARATION

IZ

Complete the following statements:

1. X-rays are one type of _____ wave.

2. The wave length of x-rays averages about _____ inch.

3. Unlike visible light, x-rays cannot be focused by means of _____ .

4. The negatively charged particles of atoms are called _____ .

5. The energy released when x-rays are created is about ____ percent heat and ____ percent x-radiation.

6. Positive poles are called _____ ; negative poles are called _____ .

7. Another name for an x-ray film is a _____ .

8. X-rays are not photographs but are essentially a record of _____ .

9. The more opaque tissue of the body will _____ a high proportion of x-rays and will therefore show as _____ areas on x-ray films.

10. The medical specialty dealing with x-rays and radioactive substances is _____ , and a specialist in the field is called a _____ .

1. Which of the following would be included in instructions to a patient scheduled for an upper G-I series?
   a. Nothing to eat after midnight before the test.
   b. No smoking the day of the test.
   c. Discontinuance of regularly taken medication if the doctor so indicates.
   d. Nothing to drink after midnight before the test—not even swallowing water after brushing teeth. _____

2. Which of the following would be included in instructions to a patient scheduled for a lower G-I series?
   a. No smoking the day of the test.
   b. Castor oil the day before the test.
   c. No food or water for 12 hours preceding the test.
   d. An enema several hours before the test. _____

3. An isotope is an element that:
   a. has the same atomic structure as another element.
   b. has the same atomic weight as another element.
   c. is always in the process of radioactive decay.
   d. is made up of atoms that have the same number of protons as another element, but a different number of neutrons.

   _____

4. Radionuclides are:
   a. stable elements.
   b. isotopes of an element that are radioactive.
   c. radiopaque.
   d. isotopes of an element that are stable.

   _____

5. "Half-life" is a means of measuring:
   a. radioactivity.
   b. the rate of decay for a radioactive material.
   c. the concentration of radionuclides in body tissue.
   d. human life expectancy.

   _____

6. Which of the following are correct statements?
   a. The effects of x-ray exposure are cumulative.
   b. The radiation absorbed from a single x-ray of the chest is about 10 percent of probable total radiation absorbed from natural sources in a year's time.
   c. The fetus is most susceptible to x-ray damage during the first trimester.
   d. Patients should be asked whether previous x-rays exist that might serve the current purpose.

   _____

C. 1. Name four special properties of x-rays.

   1. _____

   2. _____

   3. _____

   4. _____

2. Name three basic ways in which x-radiation is used in the diagnosis of medical problems.

   1. _____ 2. _____ 3. _____

3. Name four x-ray examinations that require the use of contrast media.

   1. _____ 3. _____

   2. _____ 4. _____

4. List the types of electromagnetic waves in descending order of wave length.

   1. _____ 4. _____ 6. _____

   2. _____ 5. _____ 7. _____

   3. _____

5. Name four body areas particularly sensitive to x-radiation.

1. _____   4. _____

2. _____   _____

3. _____

6. List four factors that can be harmful to unprocessed x-ray film while in storage.

1. _____   4. _____

2. _____   _____

3. _____

7. Name the four parts of the digestive tract that are examined in an upper G-I series.

1. _____   3. _____

2. _____   4. _____

8. Name the two parts of the digestive tract that are examined in a lower G-I series.

1. _____   2. _____

9. In order to be certain that no fetus is endangered by x-radiation, a general rule for taking x-rays on women of childbearing age is to schedule such work only at what times?

_____

10. What three items of identification should be on each x-ray film?

1. _____   2. _____   3. _____

For each definition below, select the term that best matches it from the column at the right. Write the term you select in the answer column.

DEFINITION	ANSWER	TERM
1. Procedure for viewing movement of internal organs	1. _____	a. cholecystogram
2. System of making radiographs of separate planes of tissue	2. _____	b. contrast media
3. Process using magnetic forces to produce images of internal tissue	3. _____	c. fluoroscopy
4. Radiograph of gallbladder	4. _____	d. mammogram
5. Radiograph of kidney	5. _____	e. nuclear magnetic resonance

6. Radiograph of breast   6. _____   f. pyelogram

7. Unit for measuring x-ray   7. _____   g. rem
   absorption

8. Unit for measuring absorption 8. _____   h. rad
   of ionizing radiation from
   any source

9. Radiopaque material used in   9. _____   i. scattered
   x-ray examination of internal   radiation
   organs

10. Deflected x-rays that may be 10. _____   j. tomography
    absorbed by x-ray technician

PRACTICE AND PROJECTS

A. What could you do to protect yourself from scattered radiation if you were
   required to assist patients while they were being x-rayed?

   _____

   What could you do to determine how much radiation exposure you were being
   subjected to?

   _____

   _____

B. Subject to the doctor's approval, what might you say to a patient to reassure
   him or her about the safety features of x-ray equipment?

   _____

   _____

   _____

   _____

   _____

20

THE DOCTOR PRESCRIBES TREATMENT

Complete the following sentences.

1. Of the various classifications of diseases, _____ are probably the most common.

2. A complex of symptoms that characterizes a particular ailment is referred to as a _____.

3. Another word for tumor is _____ which means new growth.

4. A suffix which is the medical designation for tumor is _____.

5. The two main classifications of tumors are _____ and _____.

6. Malignant tumors are generally called _____.

7. Infections are a type of disease caused by the invasion of the body by pathogenic _____.

8. A lymphoma is a _____ of the _____ tissue.

9. A blood condition in which there is an excessive number of red blood cells is called _____, whereas a condition of too few red blood cells is called _____.

10. Hemophelia is a blood ailment affecting only _____.

11. Another name for the pituitary gland is the _____.

12. The _____ glands are sometimes referred to as ductless since they secrete directly into the circulatory system.

13. The secretions of the ductless glands are _____.

14. Pathological conditions present at birth are called _____ _____.

15. A disease that lasts only a few days and is severe is described as _____;

    a disease that continues over a long period of time is described as _____.

B. 1. Name the endocrine glands.

1. _____   5. _____

2. _____   6. _____

3. _____   7. _____

4. _____

2. List four degenerative diseases.

1. _____   3. _____

2. _____   4. _____

3. Name two classifications of diseases of the mind in order of seriousness.

1. _____   2. _____

4. In treating a disease involving a painful inflammation, what two objectives would the doctor pursue?

1. _____

2. _____

5. Name the five ways in which surgery may be performed.

1. _____   4. _____

2. _____   5. _____

3. _____

6. Name five forms of treatment and give the definition for each.

TREATMENT   **DEFINITION**

1. _____   1. _____

2. _____   2. _____

                                   _____

3. _____   3. _____

   _____

4. _____   4. _____

                                   _____

5. _____   5. _____

                                   _____

144

7. List four general functions that the assistant might perform to help the physician during treatment of a patient.

1. _____

2. _____

3. _____

4. _____

For each definition below, select the term that best matches it from the column at the right. Write the term you select in the answer column.

DEFINITION	ANSWER	TERM
1. A defense reaction of the body frequently with local redness and swelling	1. _____	a. clinical
2. Disease conditions have passed but are expected to return	2. _____	b. subclinical
3. Disease conditions have lessened	3. _____	c. latent
4. Very slight case	4. _____	d. exacerbation
5. Clearly distinguishable symptoms	5. _____	e. remission
6. Greatly increased seriousness of a disease	6. _____	f. inflammation

PRACTICE AND PROJECTS

Look up the following words related to diseases and write a definition using your own words.

1. Dysfunction 1. _____

2. Asymptomatic 2. _____

3. Etiology 3. _____

4. Metastasis 4. _____

5. Somatic 5. _____

6. Prosthesis 6. _____

7. Idiopathic 7. _____

8. Endogenous 8. _____

9. Exogenous 9. _____

10. Adenoma   10._____

B. Use the "Current Medical Information and Terminology" manual to look up CYSTITIS
    ACUTE. Write down: (1) the name of the bacteria that most frequently causes
    this disease; (2) the symptoms; and (3) the prognosis.

    1._____

    2._____

    _____

    3._____

CHAPTER 21

MEDICATIONS

A. Complete the following statements:

1. The basic federal statute regulating medications is the _____
    _____.

2. The above law is administered by the _____.

3. The legally recognized compendium of medical substances is _____
    _____.

4. The federal law closely controlling the manufacture, distribution, and dis-
    pensing of narcotics and other so-called dangerous drugs is the _____
    _____ of 1970, which is administered by the _____
    _____.

5. When the trade name of a drug is registered, it is marked with the symbol
    _____.

6. A solution consists of at least two substances: the dissolved material,
    which is called the _____, and the material in which dissolution
    takes place, which is called the _____.

7. Registration to dispense controlled substances must be renewed each _____.

8. Drugs that require a prescription are identified in the Physician's Desk
    Reference by the symbol _____.

9. Prescriptions which may not be refilled are those for Schedule _____ con-
    trolled substances.

10. A drug in the Physicians' Desk Reference which is identified with the symbol
    Ⓘ is a _____ controlled substance.

11. A drug that affects a variety of organ systems is said to have _____
    effects.

B. From the items listed under each question, select the correct answer. Write the corresponding letter in the answer space.

1. To be legally qualified to administer, dispense, or prescribe controlled substances, a physician must be:
   a. registered with the Drug Enforcement Administration.
   b. registered with the U.S. Treasury.
   c. licensed to practice medicine.
   d. licensed by the state and registered with the Drug Enforcement Administration.
   _____

2. When ordering supplies of Schedule II drugs:
   a. a copy of each order must be retained on file for five years.
   b. official order forms from the Drug Enforcement Administration must be used.
   c. preprinted prescription forms should be used.
   d. the proper drug administration office must be notified.
   _____

3. Written records must be kept for:
   a. each instance when the doctor administers a narcotic drug.
   b. each instance when the doctor dispenses a narcotic drug.
   c. each instance of prescribing a narcotic drug.
   d. each instance of dispensing a drug sample.
   _____

4. A prescription for a Schedule IV controlled substance may be refilled as follows:
   a. five times within the 6 months following original date.
   b. at the discretion of a qualified pharmacist.
   c. four times within the 4 months following original date.
   d. by the medical assistant if the doctor has written the drug on the patient's chart.
   _____

5. If a container of medication were found without a label, you would:
   a. attach a new label if you think you know what the medication is.
   b. identify the medication from pictures in the "Physicians' Desk Reference" and apply a new label.
   c. discard the contents of the container.
   d. ask the physician to identify the medication and apply a new label.
   _____

C. 1. To prevent errors in the handling of medicines, there is a common rule for triple-checking which the medical assistant should always follow. List the three times when the medical assistant should check the label to be certain the medicine is the one designated by the doctor.

   1. _____

   2. _____

   3. _____

2. List three precautions the medical assistant may take to minimize the possibility of addicts obtaining narcotics improperly from the doctor.

   1. _____

2.

_____

_____

3.

_____

_____

3. List three publications that are commonly used drug references other than the one in question A-3.

1. _____

2. _____

3. _____

4. List the information that must be included on prescriptions for controlled substances.

1. _____

2. _____

3. _____

4. _____

5. _____

6. _____

7. _____

5. Instructions for taking medicine are sometimes written in abbreviated form such as t.i.d., which means "three times daily." Fill in the abbreviations for the following instructions.

1. Daily   _____   6. At bedtime   _____

2. Twice a day   _____   7. Every hour   _____

3. Four times a day _____   8. Immediately   _____

4. Before meals   _____   9. As desired   _____

5. After meals   _____   10. When required   _____

6. Explain in your own words the meaning of (1) prescribing medication; (2) administering medication; and (3) dispensing medication.

_____

_____

_____

149

_____

_____

_____

_____

_____

_____

7. Describe briefly the four processes that generally occur as a drug moves through the body.

1. _____

2. _____

3. _____

4. _____

8. Show what number of parts of solute and solvent would be mixed to make the following solutions:

	SOLUTION	PARTS OF SOLUTE	PARTS OF SOLVENT
a.	10%	_____	_____
b.	5%	_____	_____
c.	2%	_____	_____
d.	1:10	_____	_____
e.	1:4	_____	_____
f.	1:50	_____	_____

D. 1. Match the following types of drugs with their effects by writing the correct drug in the answer column.

DRUG EFFECT	ANSWER	TYPE OF DRUG
1. Inhibits growth of bacteria	1. _____	a. analgesic
2. Destroys bacteria without harm to tissue	2. _____	b. anesthetic
3. Promotes ejection of phlegm from air passage	3. _____	c. antibiotic
4. Promotes vomiting	4. _____	d. antidote

150

5. Causes loss of feeling   5._____   e. astringent

6. Promotes urination   6._____   f. antiseptic

7. Counteracts poison   7._____   g. diuretic

8. Relieves pain   8._____   h. emetic

9. Induces sleep   9._____   i. expectorant

10. Contracts tissue   10._____   j. hypnotic

2. Match the following methods of administering medication with their descriptions by writing the correct method in the answer column.

DESCRIPTION	ANSWER	METHOD
1. Introduction of liquid through the skin	1._____	a. buccal
2. Rubbing an ointment into the skin	2._____	b. injection
3. Applying directly to the skin	3._____	c. instillation
4. Absorption through the mucous membranes under the tongue	4._____	d. inunction
5. Introduction of a liquid drop by drop	5._____	e. oral
6. Passed through the gastric tract	6._____	f. sublingual
7. Absorption through the mucous membranes of gums and cheek	7._____	g. topical

3. Match the following metric terms or quantities with their definitions by writing the correct terms in the answer column.

DEFINITION	ANSWER	TERM OR QUANTITY
1. Basic unit of weight	1._____	a. centimeter
2. Basic unit of volume	2._____	b. gram
3. Basic unit of length	3._____	c. 1000 grams
4. One-thousandth of a gram	4._____	d. 100° Celsius
5. 1000 grams	5._____	e. kilogram
6. One-hundredth of a meter	6._____	f. liter
7. One-thousandth of a meter	7._____	g. meter

8. One-thousandth of a liter   8._____   h. milligram

9. Approximate weight of a liter   9._____   i. milliliter
   of water

10. Boiling point of water at sea   10._____   j. millimeter
    level

4. Match the following measuring units with the approximate quantities shown
   and write the correct unit in the answer column.

QUANTITIES	ANSWER	MEASURING UNIT
1. 1 drop	1._____	a. grain
2. 15 drops	2._____	b. gram
3. 60 drops	3._____	c. ounce (avoirdupoi
4. 3 teaspoons	4._____	d. teaspoon
5. 28 grams	5._____	e. tablespoon

PRACTICE AND PROJECTS

A. Describe how you would prepare one liter of a 1:5 solution of hydrogen peroxide
   using a 100 percent concentration of hydrogen peroxide solute and sterile water

_____

_____

B. Your doctor dispenses medication to patients and charges for this service. You
   are instructed to dispense Lomotil tablets to a patient to cover seven days wit
   directions to take 2 tablets q.i.d. for three days and 1 tablet t.i.d. for four
   days, and to call the doctor when diarrhea is controlled. Describe in your own
   words how you would carry out these instructions.

_____

_____

_____

_____

_____

_____

_____

_____

CHAPTER 22

INJECTIONS

Complete the following sentences:

1. The term hypodermic may be broken down into "hypo" meaning _____ and "derma" meaning _____ .

2. For intramuscular injections, the needles are _____ in length and have _____ lumens than the needles used in subcutaneous injections.

3. The person giving an intramuscular injection in the buttocks must be very careful to select a site well removed from the _____ nerve.

4. Allergy testing frequently makes use of _____ injections.

5. A type of injection sometimes used in the treatment of arthritis is called an _____ injection.

6. Injections into a fracture are usually for the purpose of producing local _____ .

7. The seal of a vial is wiped with _____ before a needle is inserted to withdraw medication.

8. When inserting a needle during a subcutaneous or intradermal injection, the bevel of the needle should be _____ .

From the items under each statement or question, select the correct answer and write the corresponding letter in the answer space.

1. As a rule a patient receiving an injection is likely to experience the most pain:
    a. when the needle is in its deepest position.
    b. just as the medication is beginning to enter the tissue.
    c. when the needle is penetrating the skin.
    d. when the needle is being withdrawn.   _____

2. Why is it desirable to inject a solution with a slow, steady push on the plunger of the syringe?
   a. The reaction of the patient to the medication will be less severe.
   b. The medication will push aside the tissues gradually with less trauma and discomfort to the patient.
   c. The body will absorb the medication more gradually.
   d. None of the medication will escape around the needle. _____

3. An ampul is discarded:
   a. after a single dose is withdrawn.
   b. after all medication has been used.
   c. after the neck has been broken off.
   d. when empty. _____

4. Vials are designed to hold enough medication for:
   a. a single dose only.
   b. multiple doses only.
   c. either single or multiple doses.
   d. as many doses as required for a course of treatment. _____

5. Why is air injected into a vial before medication is withdrawn?
   a. The air serves as replacement for the medication to be withdrawn.
   b. To assure that there are no air bubbles in the solution to be injected
   c. To purge the lumen of the needle.
   d. To aerate the medication. _____

6. If you had just loaded a syringe and had to put it down on a tray because the patient was not ready, how would you assure continued sterile conditions for the injection?
   a. Tilt the syringe so that the needle does not come in contact with anything.
   b. Cover the needle with cotton moistened with alcohol.
   c. Replace the needle protector.
   d. Cover the syringe and needle with a towel. _____

7. When inserting a needle for intramuscular injection, it is best to have the skin stretched taut at the injection site because:
   a. penetration will be faster and so less painful.
   b. bleeding will be less likely.
   c. the patient will be less inclined to jerk away.
   d. there is less chance of breaking the needle. _____

8. In preparation for an injection, the patient should be instructed to relax and avoid tensing of the muscles so that:
   a. the needle will penetrate more easily.
   b. the medication will be deposited with less stress to the tissues.
   c. the medication will react more quickly.
   d. both a and b above. _____

C. 1. List four conditions when it would be preferable to administer medication by injection rather than orally.

   1. _____

   2. _____

3. _____

4. _____

   _____

2. Give four examples of risks to the patient that the medical assistant should
   be aware of when an injection is being administered.

   1. _____

   2. _____

   3. _____

   4. _____

3. List two conditions that could result in infection from an injection.

   1. _____

   2. _____

4. Name five locations in the body into which medications are injected and
   give the name for each type of injection.

   LOCATION   **NAME OF INJECTION**

   1._____   1._____

   2._____   2._____

   3._____   3._____

   4._____   4._____

   5._____   5._____

   _____   _____

   _____   _____

5. Name three usable sites for subcutaneous injections, listing the most
   common one first.

   1. _____

   2. _____

   3. _____

   _____

6. Name three uses for injections into a vein.

1. _____

2. _____

3. _____

7. Name two usable sites for intradermal injections.

1. _____

2. _____

8. List two special procedures that may be used to lessen the chance that injected medication will leak from the injection site.

1. _____   2. _____

9. Give two reasons why a disposable needle and syringe should be destroyed and safely disposed of after an injection.

1. _____

2. _____

10. Name four principal sites for intramuscular injection and identify the muscles penetrated.

LOCATION	MUSCLES
1. _____	1. _____
2. _____	2. _____
3. _____	3. _____
4. _____	4. _____

D. In the left-hand column below, there are eight sets of phrases, numbers, and words that relate to three types of injections. Write the appropriate word, phrase, or number under each type of injection.

	TYPES OF INJECTIONS		
	SUBCUTANEOUS	INTRAMUSCULAR	INTRADERMA
1. Manipulation of skin			
a. Pull skin down from site			
b. Spread skin away from site	_____	_____	_____
c. Raise skin by pinching	_____	_____	_____
2. Angle of injection			
a. 90°			
b. 30° - 45°	_____	_____	_____
c. 10° - 15°			

	SUBCUTANEOUS	INTRAMUSCULAR	INTRADERMAL
3. Approximate gauge of needle 　a. 23 　b. 25 　c. 27	_____	_____	_____
4. Approximate length of needle 　a. ½ inch 　b. ⅝ inch 　c. 1¼ inch	_____	_____	_____
5. Type of injectable 　a. Allergen 　b. Aqueous 　c. Oil base	_____	_____	_____
6. Sites 　a. Gluteus maximus 　b. Inner lower arm 　c. Back of upper arm	_____ _____	_____ _____	_____ _____
7. Tissue where injectable is deposited 　a. Muscle 　b. Adipose 　c. Dermis	_____	_____	_____
8. Relative displacement of tissue by injectable 　a. Least 　b. Intermediate 　c. Most	_____	_____	_____

RACTICE AND PROJECTS

. Describe in your own words the steps you would take to prepare an area of skin for an injection.

_____

_____

_____

_____

_____

. List the steps you would take to load a syringe with 1 ml of medication contained in a vial.

1. _____

2. _____

3. _____

4. _____

5. _____

6. _____

7. _____

8. _____

9. _____

C. You have just fully inserted a needle for an intramuscular injection. Explain how you would be certain you had not entered a vein.

_____

_____

_____

What steps would you take if you had entered a vein?

_____

_____

_____

D. What special steps would you take to give an injection by the Z-track method?

_____

_____

_____

E. You are to prepare a tray for the doctor to give an injection using a disposable needle/cartridge unit. Describe what steps you would take.

_____

_____

_____

_____

_____

_____

158

. On the following figure, draw lines to indicate the four quadrants of each buttock and shade the areas where intramuscular injections should be given.

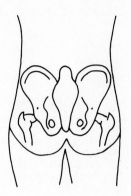

23

DIET—NUTRITIONAL PRINCIPLES

Complete the following sentences.

1. Those amino acids that are required for proper human nutrition and that cannot be manufactured within the body are referred to as _____ in our diet and must be obtained from _____.

2. When a food contains all the amino acids that the body cannot produce within itself, such food is rated high in _____.

3. In comparison with foods of animal origin, plant foods generally have _____ protein value.

4. _____ are the type of plant food rated highest in protein value.

5. Starch is reduced to _____ in the process of digestion.

6. An important carbohydrate of animal origin is _____.

7. Our common table sugar is called _____.

8. The main sources of cellulose in the diet are _____ and _____.

9. For proper nutrition, vitamins C and B (the complex), which are _____ soluble, must be included in the diet every _____.

10. The Calorie used in diet planning is described as the _____ Calorie and is the energy required to raise the temperature of one _____ of water one degree Celsius.

11. The number of Calories per gram is approximately _____ in carbohydrates, _____ in proteins, and _____ in fats.

12. When caloric intake is greater than that consumed, the excess is _____ mostly in the form of _____. One consequence is that body weight _____.

13. The basic nutritional guideline used by health professionals is a publication of the Food and Nutrition Board of the National Academy of Sciences entitled _____ which is designated by the acronym _____. The nutritional recommendations of the Food and Drug Administration used for food labeling are called the _____ _____, known by the acronym _____.

14. Saturated fats in the diet appear to _____ cholesterol, while unsaturated fats in the diet appear to _____ cholesterol.

15. Unsaturated fats generally contain less _____ than saturated fats.

16. Minerals make up approximately _____ percent of body tissue.

17. At least ____ minerals are regarded as essential for proper human nutritio

18. Water makes up approximately _____ of the body's weight.

B. From the items following each statement, select the correct one. Write the corresponding letter in the answer space.

1. Hydrogenation is a process of:
   a. removing hydrogen from a substance.
   b. liquifying a solid fat.
   c. adding hydrogen to liquid fat to make it more solid.
   d. making a fat unsaturated.   _____

2. In diet instructions an exchange food is one that may be substituted for a food printed on the basic diet list. Compared to the food in the diet, an exchange food is one that:
   a. has approximately the same calories, carbohydrates, proteins, and fats.
   b. has approximately the same taste.
   c. tastes different.
   d. has approximately the same caloric value.   _____

3. A fat controlled diet is one that:
   a. is used in the prevention and treatment of cardiovascular disease.
   b. excludes foods containing cholesterol.
   c. excludes foods containing unsaturated fats.
   d. is made up primarily of foods with low caloric value.   _____

4. Cholesterol in the body is derived from:
   a. foods of the meat group only.
   b. foods of all four of the basic food groups.
   c. foods only.
   d. synthesis within the body as well as foods.   _____

5. In planning a "low calorie" diet, one would:
    a. reduce caloric intake.
    b. increase body activities that use calories.
    c. aim for fewer calories in the diet than are used by body activities.
    d. aim for a balance between calories taken in and calories used
        by body activities.   _____

6. When planning a "bland" diet, one would:
    a. eliminate whole grain products.
    b. utilize fresh fruits and vegetables.
    c. eliminate dairy products.
    d. utilize sherbets for desserts.   _____

7. When planning a "sodium restricted" diet, one would minimize the use of:
    a. salami.
    b. antacids.
    c. softened water.
    d. all of the above.   _____

8. Fat controlled diets are primarily aimed at:
    a. reducing weight.
    b. reducing blood pressure.
    c. controlling blood lipids.
    d. eliminating cholesterol in the diet.   _____

1. Name the six classifications of food that are regarded as essential to good
    health in humans.

    1. _____   4. _____

    2. _____   5. _____

    3. _____   6. _____

2. Name five foods of animal origin that have high protein value.

    1. _____   4. _____

    2. _____   5. _____

    3. _____

3. Name the three types of food classified as carbohydrates.

    1. _____   2. _____   3. _____

4. List four fat-soluble and two water-soluble vitamins.

    FAT SOLUBLE   **WATER SOLUBLE**

    1. _____   1. _____

    2. _____   2. _____

    3. _____

    4. _____

163

5. Describe three functions of water that make it an essential part of the diet

    1. _____

    2. _____

    3. _____

6. List four ways in which calories are used by the body.

    1. _____

    2. _____

    3. _____

    4. _____

7. Name the four basic food groups in the Daily Food Guide of the U.S. Department of Agriculture.

    1. _____   3. _____

    2. _____   4. _____

8. Name the elements that make up the following foods:

                                            ELEMENTS

    1. Carbohydrates   _____

    2. Fats   _____

    3. Proteins   _____

9. All vitamins are obtainable from foods. Name two vitamins that also are available to the body by other means and describe the process.

        VITAMIN   **NON-DIETARY SOURCE**

    1. _____   _____

    2. _____   _____

D. 1. Select the food item that matches each of the following definitions and writ the correct item in the answer column.

DEFINITIONS	ANSWER	FOOD ITEM
1. A simple sugar	1. _____	a. butter
2. A saturated fat	2. _____	b. cellulose
3. An essential fatty acid	3. _____	c. glucose
4. An essential amino acid	4. _____	d. lactose
5. Digestible polysaccharide	5. _____	e. linoleic aci
6. Sugar contained in milk	6. _____	f. starch
7. Source of roughage	7. _____	g. tryptophan

2. Select the vitamin that matches the following functions and write your answer in the answer column.

FUNCTION	ANSWER	VITAMIN
1. Regulates calcium and phosphorus metabolism	1. _____	a. vitamin A
2. Promotes blood clotting	2. _____	b. vitamin B complex
3. Promotes good vision	3. _____	c. vitamin C
4. Involved in formation of connective tissue	4. _____	d. vitamin D
5. Aids muscle, nerve, and metabolic functions	5. _____	e. vitamin K

3. Select the vitamin that matches its alternative name and write your answer in the answer column.

ALTERNATIVE NAME	ANSWER	VITAMIN
1. Ascorbic acid	1. _____	a. vitamin B1
2. Nicotinic acid	2. _____	b. vitamin B2
3. Thiamine	3. _____	c. vitamin B6
4. Riboflavin	4. _____	d. vitamin B12
5. Pyridoxine	5. _____	e. vitamin C
6. Cyanobalamin	6. _____	f. Niacin

4. Select the mineral that matches the following functions in the human system and write your answers in the answer column.

FUNCTION	ANSWER	MINERAL
1. Involved in release of calcium from bone for use elsewhere	1. _____	a. calcium
2. Essential for production of thyroid hormone	2. _____	b. fluoride
3. Gives structural strength to bones	3. _____	c. iodine
4. Involved in water and electrolyte balance	4. _____	d. iron
5. Combines with protein to form hemoglobin	5. _____	e. magnesium
6. Protects against dental caries	6. _____	f. potassium

RACTICE AND PROJECTS

. Explain in your own words how fats are useful in human nutrition.

_____

_____

_____

B. Look up, in outside reference material, six foods that rate high per unit of weight in each of the following nutrients.

PROTEIN	CALCIUM	VITAMIN C	VITAMIN BI
_____	_____	_____	_____
_____	_____	_____	_____
_____	_____	_____	_____
_____	_____	_____	_____
_____	_____	_____	_____
_____	_____	_____	_____

C. From the current "Recommended Dietary Allowances," fill in the recommended daily quantities for the following nutritional items for a 30-year-old mother who is breast feeding a month-old infant.

calories	_____	thiamin	_____
protein	_____	niacin	_____
vitamin A	_____	calcium	_____
vitamin D	_____	phosphorus	_____
vitamin C	_____	iron	_____

CHAPTER 24

SURGERY IN THE OFFICE

Complete the following statements or cross out the incorrect words.

1. Prior to any surgery, the patient should be given an understandable explanation of the anesthesia and the surgical procedure and the risks involved. It is important to have the patient sign a _____ form. The signed form should be filed in the _____ _____.

2. Anesthesia means loss of the sensation of _____ or _____. This may be achieved while a patient is either conscious or _____.

3. For the surgery performed in doctors' offices, a _____ anesthetic usually is used.

4. In addition to providing insensitivity rapidly and for an adequate length of time, a local anesthetic should also have low _____.

5. Novocain is the common name for the local anesthetic drug, _____.

6. The threadlike materials used for tying off blood vessels are called _____.

7. Sutures made of catgut would be classed as absorbable/nonabsorbable and must/need not be removed when the wound is healed.

8. Sutures made of nylon or silk would be classed as absorbable/nonabsorbable and are/are not removed when the wound is healed.

9. A suturing needle that is _____ will cause less tissue distortion.

10. The materials and medications placed directly on wounds are referred to as

    _____. They are held in place by _____ or _____.

11. The surgical destruction of tissue by means of electric sparks is called

    _____.

12. A type of adhesive tape that will not allow moisture to pass through is

    referred to as _____.

13. Adhesive tape that is applied close to a wound should be removed in a

    direction _____ the wound.

B. From the items under each statement or question, select the correct answer and
   place the corresponding letter in the answer space.

1. It is good practice to write out instructions for a patient to follow
    prior to his or her coming to the office for surgery because:
    a. patients may not be concentrating and may misunderstand verbal
        instructions.
    b. patients may forget oral instructions.
    c. a written record may be needed in any dispute over proper procedure.
    d. all of the above
                                                                        _____

2. When scheduling a surgical procedure in the office, it is important to
    question the patient about previous reactions to drugs and anesthetics
    for all of the following reasons, except:
    a. there may be indications of allergies to certain drugs.
    b. this information is needed to complete the patient's record.
    c. the doctor will then know what surgical procedures to follow.
    d. strengths and types of medication may need to be changed.
                                                                        _____

3. In surgical procedures absorbent cotton:
    a. may be used as padding between dressing and bandage.
    b. may be used as dressing directly on a wound.
    c. may be used to clean a wound.
    d. should not be used at all.

4. One reason for using an elastic bandage is that:
    a. it will stretch to cover the area to be bandaged.
    b. it can be pulled tighter than an ordinary bandage.
    c. it will give under pressure caused by swelling.
    d. it makes a neater appearance.
                                                                        _____

5. All of the following are good procedures in caring for the patient
    after surgery in the office, except:
    a. have the patient taken home immediately.
    b. have the patient rest for a period of time.
    c. make sure the patient can understand and follow
        instructions before leaving the office.
    d. instruct the person accompanying the patient to
        report adverse reactions.
                                                                        _____

6. Which of the following rules should be followed in setting up and
    maintaining a sterile field?
    a. Do not touch the inside of a sterile towel used to create the field.
    b. Do not extend arms over the field.
    c. Do not place autoclaved packages on the field.
    d. All of the above.
    e. a and b above.   _____

. 1. List five points that might be covered in the instructions given to a
       patient scheduled for surgery in the doctor's office.

    1. _____

    2. _____

    3. _____

    4. _____

    5. _____

2. List four types of medication to have ready in case of an emergency during a
    surgical procedure.

    1. _____   3. _____

    2. _____   4. _____

    List three items of equipment that also should be ready.

    1. _____   3. _____

    2. _____

3. What three essential characteristics should an anesthetic agent possess?

    1. _____

    2. _____

    3. _____

       _____

4. Two purposes served by sutures are:

    1. _____

    2. _____

       _____

5. Three methods of holding the edges of wounds closed after surgery are:

   1. _____ 2. _____ 3. _____

6. List three purposes served by dressings following surgery:

   1. _____

   2. _____

   3. _____

7. List four purposes served by bandages and adhesive tape following surgery:

   1. _____

   2. _____

   3. _____

   4. _____

8. Name four types of local anesthesia and give a brief description of each.

   ANESTHESIA   **DESCRIPTION**

   1. _____   1. _____

                                 _____

   2. _____   2. _____

                                 _____

   3. _____   3. _____

                                 _____

   4. _____   4. _____

                                 _____

9. What areas of the skin should be avoided in applying adhesive tape?

   1. _____ 3. _____

   2. _____ 4. _____

10. List five surgical procedures that might be performed in a doctor's office.

    1. _____

    2. _____

    3. _____

    4. _____

    5. _____

11. List five steps to follow in applying a roller bandage.

1. _____

2. _____

3. _____

4. _____

5. _____

PRACTICE AND PROJECTS

You are making preparations for minor surgery in a doctor's office. Based on your general knowledge of the subject:

1. Describe what you would do to prepare the operating room.

1. _____

2. _____

3. _____

4. _____

5. _____

6. _____

2. List the general types of materials and equipment you would have ready.

1. _____

2. _____

3. _____

4. _____

5. _____

6. _____

7. _____

8. _____

9. _____

10. _____

11. _____

12. _____

13. _____

B. Identify the instruments pictured below and on the following page.

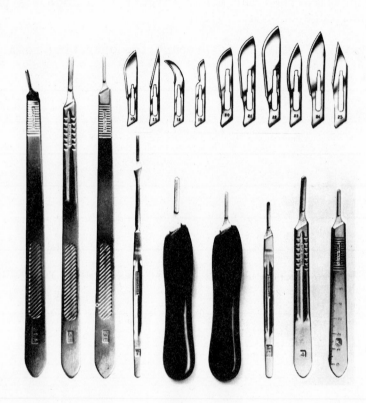

_____

_____

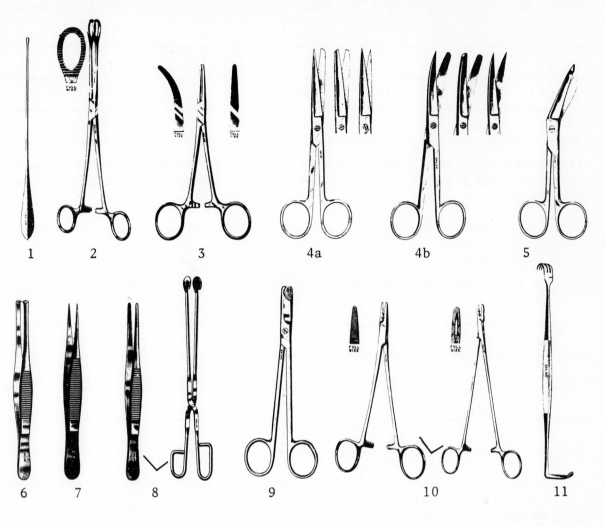

1.   6. _____

2. _____   7. _____

3. _____   8. _____

4a. _____   9. _____

4b. _____   10. _____

5. _____   11. _____

. State in your own words why it is not good practice to remove adhesive tape with a quick jerk.

_____

_____

_____

D. You are removing adhesive tape from an especially sensitive area of a patient's skin. Briefly describe what you would do to minimize pain and discomfort.

_____

_____

_____

_____

E. If you were assisting a doctor during surgery, what aspects of the patient's appearance and behavior could you observe and appropriately call to the doctor's attention?

_____

_____

F. List in order the steps you would take to put on sterile gloves.

_____

_____

_____

_____

_____

_____

_____

G. You have a patient ready and the equipment at hand to remove sutures. The sutures are of the interrupted type. List the steps you would take to remove the sutures.

_____

_____

_____

_____

_____

_____

_____

25

SPECIALIZED MEDICAL PRACTICES

1. The overall professional group that oversees and coordinates the activities of the various medical specialties is _____

   _____.

2. This group coordinates with several other leading organizations in the medical field. Name four.

   1. _____

   2. _____

   3. _____

   4. _____

3. For each specialty that is formally recognized there is a Specialty Board. List four functions of these boards.

   1. _____

   2. _____

   _____

   3. _____

   _____

   4. _____

   _____

4. A physician who is certified by a Specialty Board is called a _____.

5. Name four fields of medical practice in which the practitioners hold doctors' degrees other than Doctor of Medicine.

1. _____   3. _____

2. _____   4. _____

6. Indicate the type of work covered by each of the following dental specialties

1. Endodontia   1. _____

2. Oral surgery   2. _____

3. Orthodontia   3. _____

4. Pedontia   4. _____

5. Periodontia   5. _____

6. Prosthodontia   6. _____

7. Write out the full title of each of the following abbreviations.

1. D.D.S.   1. _____

2. D.M.D.   2. _____

3. D.O.   3. _____

4. D.P.M.   4. _____

5. M.D.   5. _____

6. O.D.   6. _____

7. D.C.   7. _____

8. A person who specializes in making eyeglasses and fitting them is called

an _____.

PRACTICE AND PROJECTS

A. Obtain a copy of the most recent edition (21st or later) of the "Directory of Medical Specialists" from your local library or from the office of a doctor who subscribes to the Directory. Using the Directory, list below those specialties for which there is a specialty board.

1. _____   3. _____

2. _____   4. _____

5. _____   15. _____

6. _____   16. _____

7. _____   17. _____

8. _____   18. _____

9. _____   19. _____

10. _____   20. _____

11. _____   21. _____

12. _____   22. _____

13. _____   23. _____

14. _____

. Look up the following specialties in a medical dictionary or other medical
reference book. In your own words, describe the field of medicine which each
one covers.

1. Immunology   1._____

                          _____

2. Oncology   2._____

                          _____

3. Nephrology   3._____

                          _____

4. Pathology   4._____

                          _____

5. Forensic pathology 5._____

                          _____

6. Neonatal   6._____

                          _____

7. Perinatal   7._____

                          _____

8. Plastic surgery   8._____

                          _____

9. Thoracic surgery 9. _____

_____

10. Geriatrics 10. _____

_____

26

ASSISTING THE SPECIALIST

A. Complete the following sentences.

1. The antibody Immunoglobulin E is abbreviated _____.

2. The type of skin testing used to identify contact allergies is _____ testing.

3. Allergies occur in about _____ percent of the population of the United States.

4. To minimize leakage, the needles used in intradermal testing are designed with _____ bevels.

5. The inability to control urine (or fecal) excretion is referred to as _____.

6. For a pelvic examination the patient usually is placed in the _____ position.

7. The instrument used for visual inspection of the vagina and cervix is a _____ _____.

8. The medical term for a whitish discharge is _____.

9. A common test to detect cancer of the cervix is the _____ test.

10. A study of cells that have been sloughed is called a _____ _____ examination.

11. When tubes within the body, such as fallopian tubes, are open, they are described as _____.

12. The presence of the hormone human chorionic gonadotropin in urine is an indication of _____.

13. Measurements of the pelvis to determine if there is sufficient capacity to permit normal birth is referred to as _____.

14. The added daily calories for a pregnant patient to allow for fetal nutrition would be approximately _____.

15. Neuritis refers to _____ of a nerve; neuralgia refers to _____ in a nerve.

16. A physician specializing in physical medicine is called a _____

17. Physical treatments prescribed by specialists in physical medicine are usually carried out by _____.

18. The use of heat produced in underlying tissues is called _____

19. The pressure within the eyeball is referred to as _____ pressure

20. The net curvature of a lens would be _____ to correct for myopia and _____ to correct for hyperopia.

21. The unit for measuring the refractive power of optic lenses is the _____

22. In a prescription for glasses, the abbreviation O.D. refers to the _____ _____ and the abbreviation O.S. refers to the _____ _____.

23. Cataract surgery involves removal of the _____ of the eye.

24. The number of bones in the human adult is _____; the number of pairs of ribs is _____.

25. Another name for joints is _____.

26. Muscles make up approximately _____ the body weight.

27. The process of restoring a fractured bone to normal position is called a _____. The process of restoring a dislocation is called a _____

28. The ear serves the body in two ways: it provides hearing and _____

29. The lowest level of intensity at which a person can hear a sound is called the hearing _____.

30. A chart showing the lowest level of intensity at which various sound frequencies can be heard is called an _____.

31. The instrument used to visually examine the larynx is the _____

32. The total number of nasal sinuses in the human body is _____.

33. The two sides of the nose are divided by a _____ consisting of bone and cartilage.

From the items under each statement or question, select the correct answer. Place the corresponding letter in the answer space.

1. The reaction time for an allergic response to take place may be:
   a. immediate.
   b. delayed.
   c. spasmodic.
   d. immediate or delayed.
   _____

2. Obstetrics covers the care of women and their offspring during:
   a. pregnancy.
   b. parturition.
   c. the puerperium.
   d. all of the above.
   e. a and b above.
   _____

3. The estimated date of confinement for a pregnant patient is November 1. Which of the following time periods would be considered normal for actual delivery?
   a. October 17 through November 1
   b. October 17 through November 15
   c. November 1 through November 15
   d. November 1
   _____

4. Which of the following would not be characteristic of a psychiatric interview?
   a. Requires minimum interruption
   b. Requires third party
   c. Is generally lengthy
   d. Can be therapeutic as well as diagnostic
   e. Development of extensive patient history
   _____

5. Which of the following would not be considered psychotherapy?
   a. oral confrontation
   b. facial expressions of disapproval
   c. hypnosis
   d. antispasmotic drugs
   _____

6. A manic-depressive state is characterized by:
   a. deep depression.
   b. mood swings between elation and depression.
   c. phobias.
   d. excessive anxieties.
   _____

7. In physical medicine, galvanic, sinusoidal, and faradic currents are used to:
   a. stimulate muscle reactions.
   b. test skin sensitivity.
   c. produce a pleasant, electrical sensation in the body.
   d. stimulate circulation of blood and lymph.
   _____

8. In carrying out ultrasonic therapy, all of the following would apply, except:
   a. the area for treatment is covered lightly with oil.
   b. the transducer is held firmly in place for the duration of the therapy.
   c. the sound-wave head is moved continuously.
   d. the treatment time will run about 10 to 15 minutes.
   _____

9. Passive exercises are performed primarily for the purpose of:
   a. aiding circulation and maintaining mobility.
   b. improving muscle tone.
   c. improving muscle strength.
   d. improving muscle tone and strength.

10. The ophthalmologic processes called refraction refer to:
    a. measurement of light absorption.
    b. a breaking down of ocular tissues.
    c. measurement of refractive errors of the eyes and
       prescribing corrective lenses.
    d. reflection of light through the eye.

11. A visual field consists of:
    a. total range of what can be seen while the head remains fixed in
       one position.
    b. total range of what can be perceived while eye is looking
       straight ahead.
    c. total range of what can be perceived with both eyes fixed.
    d. total range of what can be seen with one eye while head
       remains fixed.

12. All of the following are important rules to follow in caring for
    contact lenses except:
    a. thoroughly rinse away soap before handling lenses.
    b. carry lens container at all times.
    c. in the absence of regular whetting solutions, saliva may be used.
    d. complete all steps of insertion or removal with one eye at a time.

13. In checking lenses with a lensometer, all of the following features
    of the lens may be verified except:
    a. the axis position.
    b. the dioptic power of sphere and cylinder.
    c. the degree of prism.
    d. the tint.

14. Accommodation in ophthalmology refers to the:
    a. coordination of the eyes.
    b. adjustment of the lens for near or far vision.
    c. anesthetizing the eye prior to measurement of intra-ocular pressure.
    d. dilation of the pupil by using mydriatic drops.

15. Which of the following would not be true of a freely moving joint?
    a. The articulating surfaces are covered with cartilage.
    b. The entire joint is enclosed in a fibrous capsule.
    c. The joint is held together by tendons.
    d. The joint is lubricated with synovial fluid.

16. Which of the following would not be a function of bone?
    a. Produces red blood cells.
    b. Acts as a reservoir for calcium.
    c. Provides lubrication for joint movements.
    d. Protects internal organs.

17. An impedance audiometer is:
    a. an objective measure of middle ear mobility.
    b. a device for identifying hearing thresholds.
    c. a device that masks sound in one ear while the other is being tested.
    d. a device for producing pure tones used in hearing testing.

    _____

18. The function of the epiglottis is to cover over:
    a. the trachea when breathing.
    b. the trachea when swallowing.
    c. the larynx when breathing.
    d. the larynx when swallowing.

    _____

19. Which of the following procedures would <u>not</u> be used to stop a persistent nose-bleed?
    a. cauterization   c. packing
    b. arterial pressure point d. inflatable catheter

    _____

1. List three types of skin tests used to identify the substances causing allergic reactions.

   1. _____   3. _____

   2. _____

2. Name three ways of treating allergies.

   1. _____

   2. _____

   3. _____

      _____

3. Name four ways in which allergens may enter the body and produce allergic reactions.

   1. _____   3. _____

   2. _____   4. _____

4. Name seven parts of the female anatomy with which the gynecologist is concerned.

   1. _____   5. _____

   2. _____   6. _____

   3. _____   7. _____

   4. _____

5. List four separate steps in making a pelvic examination.

1. _____

2. _____

3. _____

4. _____

6. The microorganisms causing two of the more common types of vaginal infection are:

1. _____   2. _____

7. Name the two main parts of the central nervous system.

1. _____   2. _____

8. Name four major parts of the brain.

1. _____   3. _____

2. _____   4. _____

9. Name the two parts of the autonomic nervous system.

1. _____   2. _____

10. Both psychiatrists and psychologists treat mental illness. List three types of treatment that psychologists are not authorized to apply.

1. _____   3. _____

2. _____

11. Name nine physical agents that are utilized in the treatment of patients by doctors of physical medicine.

1. _____   4. _____   7. _____

2. _____   5. _____   8. _____

3. _____   6. _____   9. _____

12. Name three diathermy modalities.

1. _____   2. _____   3. _____

13. Name four modalities for applying superficial heat.

1. _____   3. _____

2. _____   4. _____

14. Name three types of therapeutic exercises that would require the participation of a therapist or use of a mechanical device.

1. _____ 2. _____ 3. _____

15. The two main categories of work in the specialty of ophthalmology are:

1. _____

2. _____

16. A patient being examined for visual acuity can read the 20/40 line of a Snellen chart except that one letter is missed. How would you write the results?

_____

17. Name three methods of measuring intra-ocular pressure.

1. _____ 2. _____ 3. _____

18. Name the two parts of the visual fields of each eye.

1. _____ 2. _____

19. Name two types of glaucoma and the frequently used treatment for each.

TYPE	TREATMENT
1.	1.
2.	2.

20. Name the four classifications of bones by shape and give an example of each shape.

SHAPE	EXAMPLE
1.	1.
2.	2.
3.	3.
4.	4.

21. Name the three regions that are used in the identification of specific vertebrae and give the number of vertebrae in each region.

REGION	NUMBER OF VERTEBRAE
1.	1.
2.	2.
3.	3.

22. Name the three kinds of muscles and state whether they are voluntary or involuntary.

1. _____   1. _____

2. _____   2. _____

3. _____   3. _____

23. Name the two major categories of fractures and briefly describe the outwar appearance of each.

1. _____   1. _____

2. _____   2. _____

24. Name two types of bandage rolls other than regular plaster rolls used to make casts.

1. _____   2. _____

25. Otorhinolaryngology is a combination of three special medical fields. Name the three fields and the part of the anatomy covered by each.

1. _____   1. _____

2. _____   2. _____

3. _____   3. _____

26. Name the three major parts of the ear; indicate by a √ which of these is also referred to as the labyrinth.

1. _____   _____

2. _____   _____

3. _____   _____

27. Hearing testing measures the conduction of sound in the ear through two media. Name the media and show the symbols used for each ear for each typ of sound conduction.

1. _____   1. right ear _____   left ear _____

2. _____   2. right ear _____   left ear _____

28. In addition to providing the body with a means of detecting odors, the nos conditions incoming air in three ways. Name them.

1. _____   2. _____   3. _____

D. 1. Match the following terms and definitions pertaining to allergies by writing the correct term in the answer column.

DEFINITION	ANSWER	TERM
1. A poison	1._____	a. allergen
2. A substance that neutralizes a poison	2._____	b. allergy
3. A substance that, when introduced into the body, causes production of antibodies	3._____	c. anaphylaxis
4. An antigen that causes an allergic reaction	4._____	d. antibody
5. A substance induced by exposure to an antigen	5._____	e. antigen
6. A state of hypersensitivity	6._____	f. antitoxin
7. Sensitivity to a drug	7._____	g. contactant
8. Severe allergic reactions affecting several body systems	8._____	h. intolerance
9. Protection from a disease	9._____	i. prophylaxis
10. Materials causing allergic reactions by skin contact	10._____	j. toxin

2. Match the following terms and definitions pertaining to gynecology and obstetrics by writing the correct term in the answer column.

DEFINITION	ANSWER	TERM
1. Mature male germ cells	1._____	a. colposcopy
2. Mature female germ cell	2._____	b. D and C
3. Fertilized egg	3._____	c. embryo
4. Developing human organism from conception to 8 weeks	4._____	d. endometrium
5. Developing human organism from 8 weeks to birth	5._____	e. fetus
6. Giving birth	6._____	f. hysterectomy
7. Period from delivery of placenta to resumption of menstruation	7._____	g. laparoscopy
8. Woman who has borne several viable children	8._____	h. multipara
9. Inner lining of the uterus	9._____	i. ovum
10. The pelvic floor between pubic symphysis and coccyx	10._____	j. parturition

11. Microscopic visualization   11._____   k. perineum
       of the cervix

12. Visual inspection of pelvic   12._____   l. puerperium
       organs through tube inserted
       into abdomen

13. Surgical removal of all or   13._____   m. spermatozoa
       part of the uterus

14. Removal of endometrium with   14._____   n. sterilization
       a curette   of male

15. Resection of vas deferens   15._____   o. zygote

3. Match the following terms and definitions pertaining to neurology and psychiatry by writing the correct term in the answer column.

DEFINITION	ANSWER	TERM
1. Nerve cell	1._____	a. autonomic
2. Nerve cell fiber carrying outgoing impulse	2._____	b. axon
3. Nerve cell fiber carrying incoming impulse	3._____	c. dendrite
4. Juncture of axon and dendrite	4._____	d. electroencephalography
5. Nerve system involving involuntary muscles	5._____	e. electromyograph
6. Graphic measurement of electric activity of the brain	6._____	f. encephalitis
7. Record of muscle response to electric stimulation	7._____	g. hypochondria
8. Brain inflammation	8._____	h. lobotomy
9. Excessive fear	9._____	i. neuron
10. Preoccupation with presumed illnesses	10._____	j. neuroses
11. Milder mental illnesses	11._____	k. personality disturbance
12. More severe mental illnesses	12._____	l. phobia
13. Tendency toward violent behavior	13._____	m. psychoses
14. A form of psychosurgery	14._____	n. synapse

4. Match the following terms and definitions pertaining to physical medicine by writing the correct term in the answer column.

DEFINITION	ANSWER	TERM
1. Method of applying treatment	1._____	a. conduction
2. Method of deep heating used in diathermy	2._____	b. convection
3. Method of superficial heating used in a paraffin bath	3._____	c. conversion
4. Method of heating used in hydrotherapy	4._____	d. denervated
5. Measurement of extent of joint mobility	5._____	e. effleurage
6. Light, stroking massage	6._____	f. electrotherapy
7. Kneading or friction massage	7._____	g. goniometry
8. Tapping or beating massage	8._____	h. modality
9. Low-voltage stimulation of muscles	9._____	i. petrissage
10. Having no nerve supply	10._____	j. postural drainage
11. A form of respiratory physical therapy	11._____	k. tapotement

5. Matching the following terms and definitions pertaining to instruments and materials used in the practice of ophthalmology by writing the correct term in the answer column.

DEFINITION	ANSWER	TERM
1. Used by ophthalmologist to objectively judge refractive error	1._____	a. goniolens
2. Hand-held instrument for inspecting interior of eye for defects	2._____	b. Jeager chart
3. Provides binocular microscopic examination of eye surface	3._____	c. keratometer
4. Used to view anterior chamber angle	4._____	d. lensometer
5. Used for testing distant vision	5._____	e. ophthalmoscope
6. Used for testing near vision	6._____	f. perimeter
7. Holds trial lenses for vision testing	7._____	g. phoropter

8. Measures curvature of cornea   8._____   h. retinoscope

9. Measures visual fields   9._____   i. Schiötz tono-
meter

10. Used to check refractive
characteristics of glasses   10._____   j. slit lamp

11. Measures intraocular
pressure by indentation   11._____   k. Snellen chart

6. Match the following terms and definitions pertaining to eye conditions and diseases by writing the correct term in the answer column.

DEFINITION	ANSWER	TERM
1. Visual image focuses on retina	1._____	a. astigmatism
2. Visual image focuses in front of retina	2._____	b. blepharitis
3. Visual image focuses behind retina	3._____	c. cataract
4. Part of image is in focus and part is distorted	4._____	d. conjunctiviti
5. High intra-ocular pressure damages optic nerve and retina	5._____	e. emmetropia
6. Area of visual field without sight perception	6._____	f. glaucoma
7. Inflammation of cornea	7._____	g. hordeolum
8. Inflammation of mucous membrane of the eye	8._____	h. hyperopia
9. Inflammation of eyelid margins	9._____	i. keratitis
10. Crossed eyes	10._____	j. myopia
11. A sty	11._____	k. scotoma
12. Opacity of the lens	12._____	1. strabismus

7. Match the following definitions and types of lenses by writing the correct type of lens in the answer column.

DEFINITION	ANSWER	TYPE OF LENS
1. Refracts light equally in all directions	1._____	a. compound
2. Provides more converging focus	2._____	b. concave
3. Provides more diverging focus	3._____	c. convex

4. Having convex surface on one side and concave on the other

4. _____

d. cylindrical

5. Combination of spherical and cylindrical properties in a single lens

5. _____

e. meniscus

6. Used to correct for astigmatism

6. _____

f. spherical

8. Match the following definitions and terms pertaining to the musculoskeletal system by writing the correct term in the answer column.

DEFINITION	ANSWER	TERM
1. Membrane covering bone	1. _____	a. bursa
2. Developing bone cells	2. _____	b. cartilage
3. Space within bone containing marrow	3. _____	c. foramen
4. Hole in bone for passage of blood vessels, nerves	4. _____	d. fossa
5. Depression in surface of bone	5. _____	e. insertion
6. A bone projection	6. _____	f. ligament
7. A cavity within bone	7. _____	g. medullary canal
8. Covering for joint surfaces	8. _____	h. origin
9. Fibrous cords connecting bones	9. _____	i. osteoblasts
10. Fibrous cords connecting muscle to bone	10. _____	j. periosteum
11. Sac-like structures serving to reduce friction between rubbing parts	11. _____	k. process
12. Attachment of muscle to relatively stationary bone	12. _____	l. sinus
13. Attachment of muscle to more moveable bone.	13. _____	m. tendon

9. Match the following definitions and terms pertaining to musculoskeletal deformities, injuries, and diseases by writing the correct term in the answer column.

DEFINITION	ANSWER	TERM
1. Backward thoracic spinal curvature	1. _____	a. callus
2. Forward lumbar spinal curvature	2. _____	b. comminuted
3. Lateral spinal curvature	3. _____	c. greenstick

4.	Fracture in which bone shaft is driven into bone end	4. _____	d. impacted
5.	Fracture involving several breaks and bone splinters	5. _____	e. kyphosis
6.	Fracture in which not all fibers are broken	6. _____	f. lordosis
7.	Partial dislocation	7. _____	g. orthoses
8.	First layer next to skin in making a cast	8. _____	h. osteoarthriti
9.	Braces for misaligned or poorly functioning part	9. _____	i. osteoporosis
10.	Bony tissue surrounding fracture during healing	10. _____	j. scoliosis
11.	Degenerative disease of joints	11. _____	k. stockinet
12.	Disease involving shrinkage of bone size	12. _____	l. subluxation

10. Match the following types of muscle movement with their definition. Write the correct movement in the answer column.

	DEFINITION	ANSWER	MUSCLE MOVEMENT
1.	Increases angle of joint	1. _____	a. abduction
2.	Decreases angle of joint	2. _____	b. adduction
3.	Moves appendicular bones toward the body mid-line	3. _____	c. eversion
4.	Moves appendicular bones away from body mid-line	4. _____	d. extension
5.	Turning up—e.g., the hands	5. _____	e. flexion
6.	Turning down—e.g., the hands	6. _____	f. inversion
7.	Turning out—e.g., the hands	7. _____	g. pronation
8.	Turning in—e.g., the hands	8. _____	h. supination

11. Match the following definitions and terms pertaining to otology by writing the correct item in the answer column.

	DEFINITION	ANSWER	TERM
1.	Semicircular canals, vestibule, and cochlea	1. _____	a. barotitis

2. Bones of the middle ear   2._____   b. cerumen

3. Ringing in ears when no sound   3._____   c. decible
is present

4. Inflammation of ear caused by   4._____   d. Hertz (Hz)
air pressure change

5. Bone growth that impairs   5._____   e. labyrinth
function of stapes

6. Disease causing dizziness,   6._____   f. Meniere's
deafness, tinnitus

7. Dizziness   7._____   g. nystagmus

8. Rhythmic eye movements   8._____   h. ossicles

9. Unit measuring sound intensity   9._____   i. otosclerosis

10. Cycles per second   10._____   j. tinnitus

11. Ear wax   11._____   k. vertigo

12. Match the following definitions and terms pertaining to rhinology and
larynogology by writing the correct term in the answer column.

DEFINITION	ANSWER	TERM
1. External openings of the nose	1._____	a. adenoid hypertrophy
2. Scroll-shaped bones covered with mucous membrane	2._____	b. adenoids
3. Hairs that filter air in the nose	3._____	c. cilia
4. Oval lymph masses at back of oropharynx	4._____	d. epistaxis
5. Lymphoid tissue in nasopharynx	5._____	e. larynx
6. Extends from the soft palate to the top of the epiglottis	6._____	f. nares
7. Tubular structure containing vocal chords	7._____	g. nasal conchae
8. Nose bleed	8._____	h. oropharynx
9. Enlarged lymph tissue that may block eustachian tube	9._____	i. palatine tonsils
10. Inflammation of nasal passages	10._____	j. rhinitis

PRACTICE AND PROJECTS

A. Briefly describe the procedure for making the following two types of allergy tests.

    1. Prick Test

_____

_____

_____

_____

_____

_____

    2. Scratch Test

_____

_____

_____

_____

_____

_____

_____

B. Explain briefly why patch tests have clear plastic over the material being tested for possible allergic reaction.

_____

_____

C. Briefly describe the following two infertility tests for women:

    1. Tubal insufflation

_____

_____

_____

2. Hysterosalpingography

_____

_____

_____

_____

Fill in the following table covering the three stages of labor.

| | BEGINNING | ENDING | AVERAGE DURATION | |
			PRIMAPARAS	MULTIPARAS
1ST STAGE				
2ND STAGE				
3RD STAGE				

Calculate the estimated date of confinement for the following pregnant patients.

1. First day of last menstrual period was March 1. _____

2. First day of last menstrual period was April 7. _____

You are asked to watch a patient who is being given shorwave diathermy. What instructions would you give the patient to ensure that the treatment is not excessive?

_____

_____

_____

_____

List the steps you would take to instill drops in a patient's eye.

_____

_____

_____

_____

_____

_____

_____

_____

_____

H. List some of the things you might do to assist an orthopedist apply a plaster cast.

_____

_____

_____

_____

_____

_____

_____

I. Briefly describe how crutches should be used when one leg is not to touch the floor.

_____

_____

_____

_____

J. Outline the steps you would take to irrigate a patient's right ear.

1. _____

2. _____

3. _____

4. _____

5. _____

6. _____

7.   _____

8.   _____

9.   _____

10. _____

11. _____

12. _____

13. _____

14. _____

     _____

     _____

. A patient has just been treated for a nose bleed that was difficult to control.
What are some of the self-care measures you might remind the patient to observe?

_____

_____

_____

_____

_____

L. Study the sketch below. Write in the correct term for each part indicated by an arrow.

a._____

b._____

c._____

d._____

e._____

f._____

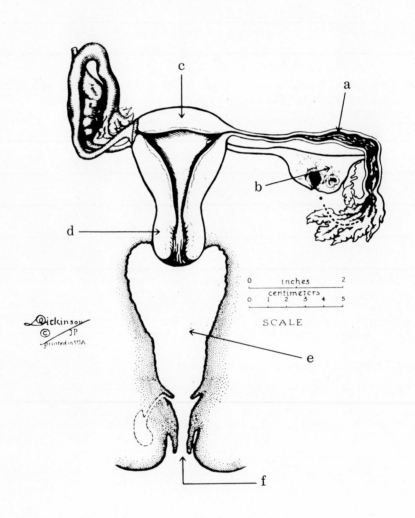

4. Study the cross section of the eye shown below; fill in the names of those parts of the eye that are not identified in the drawing. Refer to Figure 26-23 in the text.

1. _____   7. _____

2. _____   8. _____

3. _____   9. _____

4. _____   10. _____

5. _____   11. _____

6. _____

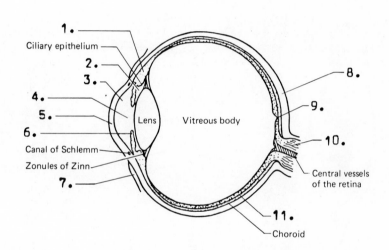

N. Study the drawing of the ear shown below; fill in the names of those parts of the ear that are not identified in the drawing. Refer to Figure 26-40 in the text.

1. _____   6. _____

2. _____   7. _____

3. _____   8. _____

4. _____   9. _____

5. _____   10. _____

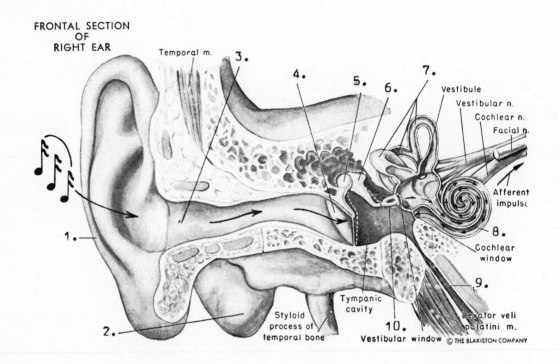

FRONTAL SECTION
OF
RIGHT EAR

Temporal m.

Vestibule
Vestibular n.
Cochlear n.
Facial n.

Afferent impulse

Cochlear window

Tympanic cavity

Styloid process of temporal bone

Levator veli palatini m.

Vestibular window © THE BLAKISTON COMPANY

Study the drawing of the pharynx and larynx shown below; fill in the names of those parts that are not identified in the drawing. Refer to Figure 26-46 in the text.

1. _____   6. _____

2. _____   7. _____

3. _____   8. _____

4. _____   9. _____

5. _____

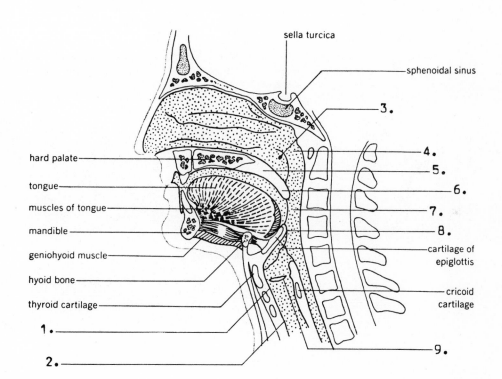

CHAPTER 27

CHILDREN IN THE DOCTOR'S OFFICE

1. The following are general statements about handling children in a doctor's office. Check (√) the ones you feel represent good practice and put an (X) beside those that you feel do not.

   _____a. Speak to a child in terms he or she can understand.

   _____b. Try to have the child see things from your viewpoint.

   _____c. Gaining a child's confidence and good will are not especially helpful.

   _____d. Children in the same age group should be treated alike.

   _____e. It is better to explain that a procedure will hurt if such is likely to be the case.

   _____f. It is better to call upon a child's desire to be thought of as "grown-up" rather than threaten punishment for poor behavior.

   _____g. Truthful explanation is better than reassurances that turn out to be false.

   _____h. Firmness is necessary, but tempered with kindness.

   _____i. Commands are a better means of getting cooperation than requests.

   _____j. The individual personality of each child should be recognized.

   _____k. Children should not be mocked or made fun of regarding fears of medical examination or treatment.

   _____l. Medical treatment should never be equated with punishment.

   _____m. Children should not be asked to help with any aspect of their medical treatment.

   _____n. Preparations for examination or treatment should be completed before the child patient is present.

   _____o. It is best to move quickly in handling an infant.

_____p. It is best to recognize that a child's fear of medical treatment is reasonable and to focus on trying to help the child overcome the fear.

_____q. When an infant patient has become highly irritated in the reception room, it is best that the doctor not see the infant until it has quieted down.

_____r. For children through age 3 any undressing should be done by the parent.

_____s. Children aged 4 through 5 should be encouraged to undress and dress themselves.

2. The following list contains items for occupying the attention of young children in a doctor's reception room. Check (√) the ones you feel are good selections and put an (X) beside those you feel are not.

_____a. Coloring books   _____h. Wind-up racing car

_____b. Marbles   _____i. Darts

_____c. Ball and jacks   _____j. Frisbees

_____d. Building blocks   _____k. Jigsaw puzzle

_____e. Picture books   _____l. Soft plastic animals

_____f. Fire engine with siren   _____m. Stuffed toys with embroidered faces

_____g. Skipping rope

B. From the items under each statement, select the correct answer or answers and write the corresponding letter or letters in the answer space.

1. Indicate which of the following are characteristics of an infant.
   a. Resists giving up toys.
   b. Shows anxiety if separated from mother.
   c. Has close to 20/20 visual acuity.
   d. Should be able to understand the word "come" by 12 months.   _____

2. Which of the following are characteristics of children 1 to 3 years old?
   a. Have ability to dress themselves.
   b. Prone to temper tantrums.
   c. At 24 months may be able to indicate need to go to the toilet.
   d. At 36 months should have bladder and bowel control.   _____

3. Which of the following are characteristics of children aged 4 and 5?
   a. Anger more likely to be expressed in language.
   b. Like being center of attraction.
   c. Able to apply logic.
   d. Can follow simple directions.   _____

4. Which of the following are characteristics of children aged 6 through 12?
   a. Can think in the abstract.
   b. Can be influenced by appeals to reason.
   c. Want to be treated more as equals.
   d. Not yet interested in what happens in the office.
   _____

5. When a parent comes with a teenaged patient to the doctor's office:
   a. the parent should not be allowed in the examining room.
   b. the parents should be asked to be with the teenager during examination.
   c. if the teenager requests and the parent agrees, the teenager may be examined in private.
   d. if the teenager requests, the parent should be asked to remain in the reception room.
   _____

6. Advice to a parent regarding preparing a child for a visit to a doctor might include:
   a. to tell the child a day or more in advance in order to avoid surprise.
   b. to avoid explanations of reasons for visit.
   c. to see that the child understands that uncooperative behavior will be punished.
   d. to tell the child it is a normal part of growing up.
   _____

1. A typical schedule for periodic medical check-ups for children would be:

   1. once every _____ during the first six months.

   2. once every _____ from age 6 months to 2 years.

   3. once every _____ from age 2 to 6 years.

   4. once every _____ from age 6 years on.

2. What do the following abbreviations stand for in an immunization schedule for children?

   1. DTP _____

   2. OPV _____

   3. MMR _____

3. In completing the patient's record, the information about a vaccine or biologic used for immunization should include:

   1._____   3._____

   2._____   4._____

4. During the first four weeks after birth, the baby may be referred to as a

   newborn or _____.

5. Beginning at what age is it appropriate to provide privacy for a child who must undress for an examination?_____

6. The frequency of appointments for physical examination and inoculation of children is likely to be highest in the months of _____ and _____.

7. List three conditions that might be indications of child neglect or abuse.

1._____

2._____

3._____

_____

PRACTICE AND PROJECTS

A. You are about to take blood from the finger of a six-year-old boy. He is afrai of how much it will hurt. Describe how you would handle this situation.

_____

_____

_____

_____

_____

_____

_____

_____

B. Describe how you would wrap a sheet around an infant to restrain the child whil the doctor examines the mouth and throat.

1._____

2._____

3._____

4._____

5._____

6._____

C. Make up a standard list of questions that you might use when a parent telephones to say that a child is ill. These would be questions that the doctor would authorize you to ask if he or she were unable to take the call.

1. _____

2. _____

3. _____

4. _____

5. _____

6. _____

7. _____

D. Look up the following diseases. Write the definition in your own words, and give the common name for each.

1. Tetanus

_____

_____

_____

Common name: _____

2. Pertussis

_____

_____

_____

Common name: _____

3. Rubella

_____

_____

_____

Common name: _____

E. What suggestions might you give to a parent regarding ways to restrain a very active two-year-old while instilling eye drops?

_____

_____

_____

_____

28

ELDERLY AND
HANDICAPPED PATIENTS

1. The following are general statements about handling an elderly patient in a doctor's office. Check (√) the ones you feel represent good practice or viewpoint and put an (X) beside those you feel do not.

   _____ a. Generally go beyond what you would ordinarily do for other patients.

   _____ b. Tactfully provide any extra measure of assistance that would be helpful.

   _____ c. Keep the patients away from others as much as possible.

   _____ d. Make the patient feel as welcome as any other patient.

   _____ e. Give the patient every opportunity to make his or her own decisions.

   _____ f. Avoid talking to the patient in a patronizing manner.

   _____ g. All patients over 65 years of age will need special help.

   _____ h. It is better to be respectful of an elderly patient than to baby him or her along.

   _____ i. Assessing the special needs of each individual elderly patient is part of the medical assistant's job.

   _____ j. Encourage the patient to depend on his or her memory.

   _____ k. Do not draw attention to the fact that the patient is causing extra effort on your part.

   _____ l. Try to imagine yourself in the patient's shoes in order to understand him or her better.

   _____ m. It is not particularly helpful to slow down your conversation to match the patient's slower reaction to what is being said.

   _____ n. Emotional problems of the patient should be taken into consideration as much as the physical problems.

   _____ o. Facing up to the reasons why a patient may feel depressed is better than glossing over the problem.

_____p. Assuring privacy is less important in handling elderly patients.

_____q. Elderly patients sometimes are quite talkative, so there is no need to be alert to new information that the patient may bring out.

2. The following are general statements about handling handicapped patients in a doctor's office. Check (√) the ones you feel represent good practice or viewpoint and put an (X) beside those you feel do not.

_____a. In making appointments, the medical assistant should consider that extra time may be needed.

_____b. The medical assistant should become familiar with the specific kind of assistance each patient needs.

_____c. In the doctor's office, handicapped patients may reveal more about their difficulties than in other surroundings.

_____d. When approaching a blind person, introduce yourself promptly.

_____e. When guiding a blind person through the office, offer your arm and lead the way.

_____f. Privacy is not as important to a blind patient as to others.

_____g. The use of a little sign language will probably help a deaf patient feel more at home.

_____h. In order to save time, communications with deaf patients should be limited to the medical matters of the case.

_____i. Before helping to move a wheelchair patient, the medical assistant might ask the patient what type of lifting would not be injurious.

_____j. Persons who are blind are often better than average at remembering.

_____k. When another person brings a blind patient to the office, address questions to the other person.

_____l. Gestures and facial expressions are good ways of communicating with a deaf person.

B. Complete the following sentences or answer the questions in the space provided.

1. Approximately _____ percent of the population of the United States is 65 years of age or older.

2. Which of the senses are likely to deteriorate with old age? _____

3. In elderly persons the epithelium and subcutaneous tissue layers become

_____.

4. The muscles of elderly persons become smaller in size and _____

5. A thermometer that would give readings down to 86°F is called a _____ thermometer.

From the items under each statement or question, select the correct answer. Write the corresponding letter in the answer space.

1. If you are concerned that an elderly patient may not clearly have heard verbal instructions you have given:
   a. ask the patient to repeat the instructions to you.
   b. have the doctor repeat the instructions.
   c. do not embarrass the patient by questioning his or her ability to hear.
   d. tell the patient to listen more carefully.   _____

2. When an older patient with a failing memory appears at the office on the wrong day, which one of the following would be poor practice?
   a. Make an effort to have the doctor see the patient if only for a few minutes.
   b. Avoid any disagreement about who is in the wrong.
   c. Make out a new appointment card and review it with the patient.
   d. Make sure the patient realizes the mistake and emphasize the need to arrive on the right day next time.   _____

3. When you are questioning an older person about his or her condition and you know the patient may have difficulty remembering, which one of the following would be poor practice?
   a. If an answer seems improbable, ask the same or similar question later in the conversation and cross check.
   b. Simply ignore any answers that seem improbable.
   c. Realize that the patient may give a wrong answer if the correct answer cannot be remembered.
   d. Check an answer that seems improbable by asking the question of the person accompanying the patient.   _____

4. When receiving an elderly male patient for an office visit, which of the following questions would be inappropriate?
   a. Have you been following the doctor's instructions?
   b. Have you been a good boy?
   c. Have you been feeling well?
   d. Did you have any difficulty getting to the office today?   _____

5. If an argument develops in the office between an elderly patient and a son or daughter of the patient, which one of the following reactions would be appropriate for the medical assistant?
   a. Support the view of the patient.
   b. Call for the doctor.
   c. Remain calm and neutral.
   d. Support whichever party appears to be more right.   _____

CTICE AND PROJECTS

Describe several things you might do to help an elderly patient with a hearing deficiency understand what you say.

1. _____

211

2. _____

3. _____

4. _____

B. Your doctor-employer has a number of elderly patients who have sometimes forgotten what the doctor's instructions are. What might you suggest to help overcome this difficulty?

_____

_____

_____

_____

_____

_____

C. What would you do to break off an overly long conversation with an elderly patient who just wanted to keep talking?

_____

_____

_____

D. Your doctor is out of the office for several hours and you receive a call from a patient who is caring for her invalid 88-year-old mother. The patient says that her mother is unusually lethargic and unresponsive. The weather has been unusually cold. What questions might you ask in order to develop more information to give to the doctor?

_____

_____

_____

_____

E. In discussing health problems with elderly patients, what should you keep in mind regarding such patients' reaction to:

Pain _____

Fever _____

Drugs _____

. A deaf patient is relying on lip reading to understand what you say. What can you do to make it easier for the patient to read your lips?

_____

_____

_____

_____

_____

. A new patient calls to make an appointment. He explains that he is blind and will be coming to the office with his guide dog. What nonmedical information would you ask for in order to handle this patient satisfactorily?

_____

_____

_____

_____

_____

_____

_____

_____

MEDICAL TERMS

. For each term or phrase in the left column, select the correct abbreviation from the column on the right and write the abbreviation in the answer space in the center.

TERM	ANSWER	ABBREVIATION
1. Gram	1._____	a. ad lib
2. Grain	2._____	b. bid
3. Drop	3._____	c. db
4. Drops	4._____	d. dr
5. Dram	5._____	e. g
6. Milliliter	6._____	f. gr
7. Microliter	7._____	g. gt
8. Two times a day	8._____	h. gtt
9. Three times a day	9._____	i. Hb
10. Four times a day	10._____	j. Hg
11. At will	11._____	k. hs
12. At bedtime	12._____	l. ml
13. Decibel	13._____	m. NPO
14. Right eye	14._____	n. OD
15. Left eye	15._____	o. OS
16. Immediately	16._____	p. qid
17. Tincture	17._____	q. stat
18. Nothing by mouth	18._____	r. tid
19. Hemoglobin	19._____	s. tr
20. Mercury	20._____	t. µl

B. Write the meaning after each of the following acronyms.

1. BUN _____ 11. FEV _____

2. CBC _____ 12. HCG _____

3. CCU _____ 13. ICU _____

4. CNS _____ 14. IM _____

5. CRT _____ 15. IV _____

6. CT _____ 16. MVV _____

7. CVA _____ 17. PDR _____

8. EEG _____ 18. URI _____

9. ENT _____ 19. UTI _____

10. ESR _____ 20. VC _____

PREFIXES AND SUFFICES

A. For each of the following definitions, select the correct prefix from the right hand column and write it in the answer column.

DEFINITION	ANSWER	PREFIX
1. Toward	1._____	a. ab
2. Away from	2._____	b. ad
3. To the back	3._____	c. andro
4. To the front or abdomen	4._____	d. auto
5. Within	5._____	e. brady
6. Outside of	6._____	f. cryo
7. Around	7._____	g. dorso
8. Over	8._____	h. dys
9. Under	9._____	i. endo
10. Good	10._____	j. epi
11. Bad	11._____	k. erythro
12. Faulty	12._____	l. eu
13. New	13._____	m. exo

216

14.	Fast	14._____		n.	gyno
15.	Slow	15._____		o.	infra
16.	Large	16._____		p.	leuko
17.	Small	17._____		q.	macro
18.	Self	18._____		r.	mal
19.	Male	19._____		s.	melano
20.	Female	20._____		t.	micro
21.	White	21._____		u.	neo
22.	Black	22._____		v.	peri
23.	Red	23._____		w.	pyro
24.	Heat	24._____		x.	tachy
25.	Cold	25._____		y.	ventro

3. For each of the following definitions, select the correct suffix from the right hand column and write it in the answer column.

DEFINITIONS	ANSWER	SUFFIX
1. Surgical removal	1._____	a. algia
2. Cut into	2._____	b. ase
3. Inspection of	3._____	c. blast
4. Pain	4._____	d. cide
5. Inflammation	5._____	e. cyte
6. Deficiency	6._____	f. ectomy
7. Paralysis	7._____	g. emia
8. Tendency toward	8._____	h. iasis
9. Sudden flow	9._____	i. itis
10. Excessive flow	10._____	j. lysis
11. Consuming	11._____	k. osis
12. State or condition	12._____	l. penia
13. Suture of	13._____	m. phage
14. Setting free	14._____	n. plegia

15.	Enzyme	15._____	o.	rraphy
16.	Developing state	16._____	p.	rrhagia
17.	Cell	17._____	q.	rrhea
18.	Causing death	18._____	r.	scopy
19.	Blood	19._____	s.	tomy
20.	Condition of	20._____	t.	tropy

WORD ROOTS

A. Name the body part referred to in each of the following medical terms.

1. Arthritis _____	11. Orchiectomy _____
2. Hepatitis _____	12. Gastrectomy _____
3. Cystitis _____	13. Cholecystectomy _____
4. Phlebitis _____	14. Mastectomy _____
5. Encephalitis _____	15. Cardiology _____
6. Blepharitis _____	16. Endocrinology _____
7. Nephritis _____	17. Hematology _____
8. Hysterectomy _____	18. Rhinology _____
9. Prostatectomy _____	19. Dermatology _____
10. Oophorectomy _____	20. Intercostal _____

B. For each of the following medical terms, select the body part or tissue from the right-hand column and write it in the answer column.

MEDICAL TERM	ANSWER		BODY PART OR TISSUE
1. Acromegaly	1._____	a.	abdominal wall
2. Adenopathy	2._____	b.	bile duct
3. Aphakia	3._____	c.	bone
4. Biliary	4._____	d.	brain or diaphragm
5. Cellulitis	5._____	e.	buttocks
6. Endometrium	6._____	f.	connective tissue
7. Enteritis	7._____	g.	cornea
8. Epiglottis	8._____	h.	ductus deferens

218

9.	Gluteal	9._____	i.	glands
10.	Keratitis	10._____	j.	intestinal tract
11.	Laparotomy	11._____	k.	lens
12.	Myoma	12._____	l.	limbs, head
13.	Periosteum	13._____	m.	lungs
14.	Phrenic	14._____	n.	membrane around lungs
15.	Pleurisy	15._____	o.	muscle
16.	Pulmonary	16._____	p.	opening from kidney to ureter
17.	Pyelography	17._____	q.	cartilage at top of larynx
18.	Salpingography	18._____	r.	spleen
19.	Splenitis	19._____	s.	uterine tubes
20.	Vasectomy	20._____	t.	uterus

ᴇDICAL TERMS FOR EVERYDAY WORDS OR PHRASES

Listed below are words or phrases used in everyday language for parts of the human anatomy. Select the matching medical term from the right-hand column and write the term in the answer column.

	WORD OR PHRASE	ANSWER		MEDICAL TERM
1.	Eardrum	1._____	a.	axilla
2.	White of eye	2._____	b.	bucca
3.	Nostril	3._____	c.	carpus
4.	Cheek	4._____	d.	clavicle
5.	Jaw bone	5._____	e.	coccyx
6.	Voice box	6._____	f.	coxa
7.	Windpipe	7._____	g.	cubitus
8.	Collar bone	8._____	h.	larynx
9.	Shoulder blade	9._____	i.	mandible
10.	Breast bone	10._____	j.	naris
11.	Armpit	11._____	k.	patella
12.	Elbow	12._____	l.	phalanges

13. Wrist	13._____	m.	scapula
14. Fingers, toes	14._____	n.	sclera
15. Back bone	15._____	o.	sternum
16. Tail bone	16._____	p.	tibia
17. Womb	17._____	q.	trachea
18. Hip	18._____	r.	tympanic membrane
19. Knee cap	19._____	s.	uterus
20. Shin bone	20._____	t.	vertebral column

B. Listed below are words or phrases used in everyday language for various disorder and diseases. Select the matching medical term from the right-hand column and write the term in the answer column.

WORD OR PHRASE	ANSWER		MEDICAL TERM
1. Blood poisoning	1._____	a.	arteriosclerosis
2. Boil	2._____	b.	cerebrovascular accident
3. Common cold	3._____	c.	conjunctivitis
4. Earache	4._____	d.	coryza
5. Feverish	5._____	e.	edema
6. Hardening of the arteries	6._____	f.	emesis
7. High blood pressure	7._____	g.	epistaxis
8. Hives	8._____	h.	febrile
9. Jaundice	9._____	i.	furuncle
10. Low blood pressure	10._____	j.	hemorrhoids
11. Near sightedness	11._____	k.	herpes zoster
12. Nosebleed	12._____	l.	hordeolum
13. Piles	13._____	m.	hypertension
14. Pinkeye	14._____	n.	hypotension
15. Shingles	15._____	o.	icterus
16. Swelling	16._____	p.	myopia
17. Stroke	17._____	q.	otalgia

18. Sty	18._____	r. pertussis
19. Vomiting	19._____	s. septicemia
20. Whooping cough	20._____	t. urticaria

Listed below are words or phrases used in everyday language for various physical conditions and functions. Select the matching medical term from the right-hand column and write the term in the answer column.

WORD OR PHRASE	ANSWER	MEDICAL TERM
1. Baldness	1._____	a. adipose
2. Belching	2._____	b. alopecia
3. Bruise	3._____	c. angina
4. Change of life	4._____	d. aqueous
5. Corn	5._____	e. cerumen
6. Dizziness	6._____	f. clavus
7. Earwax	7._____	g. contusion
8. Fainting	8._____	h. crepitus
9. Fatty	9._____	i. eructation
10. Gas from rectum	10._____	j. flatus
11. Hairy	11._____	k. gustation
12. Itchy	12._____	l. hirsute
13. Pain	13._____	m. menopause
14. Paralysis	14._____	n. micturition
15. Passing gas	15._____	o. palsy
16. Ringing in ears	16._____	p. pruritic
17. Setting of fracture	17._____	q. reduction
18. Tasting	18._____	r. syncope
19. Urination	19._____	s. tinnitus
20. Watery	20._____	t. vertigo

Listed below are a variety of commonly used words or phrases for which there are medical terms. Select from the column on the right the correct medical term and write it in the answer column.

WORD OR PHRASE	ANSWER	MEDICAL TERM
1. Afterbirth	1._____	a. amnesia
2. Kidney stone	2._____	b. borborygmus
3. Eye socket	3._____	c. calculus
4. Eye lid	4._____	d. diplopia
5. Crossed eyes	5._____	e. dyspnea
6. Double vision	6._____	f. emmetropia
7. Perfect vision	7._____	g. erythema
8. Blood clot	8._____	h. hernia
9. Wart	9._____	i. orbit
10. Goiter	10._____	j. palpebra
11. Navel	11._____	k. placenta
12. Loss of memory	12._____	l. Rubella
13. Rumbling of gas in intestines	13._____	m. sclerosis
14. Labored breathing	14._____	n. stenosis
15. Rupture	15._____	o. strabismus
16. Sunburn	16._____	p. struma
17. Injury	17._____	q. thrombus
18. German measles	18._____	r. trauma
19. Hardening	19._____	s. umbilicus
20. Stricture	20._____	t. verruca

E. Listed below are additional commonly used words or phrases for which there are medical terms. Select the correct medical term from the right-hand column and write the term in the answer column.

WORD OR PHRASE	ANSWER	MEDICAL TERM
1. Scar	1._____	a. abort
2. Excess scar tissue	2._____	b. amorphous
3. Ulcer	3._____	c. ataraxic
4. Shapeless	4._____	d. cicatrix
5. Wedge-shaped	5._____	e. cuneiform

222

6.	Clubfoot	6._____	f.	hemorrhage
7.	Humpback	7._____	g.	hyperopia
8.	Swayback	8._____	h.	hypnotic
9.	Sleeping pill	9._____	i.	keloid
10.	Tranquilizer	10._____	j.	kyphosis
11.	Bleed	11._____	k.	lordosis
12.	Miscarry	12._____	l.	lues
13.	Birthmark	13._____	m.	nevus
14.	Poisonous	14._____	n.	scotoma
15.	Instep	15._____	o.	talipes
16.	Straining to move bowels	16._____	p.	tarsus
17.	Blind spot	17._____	q.	tenesmus
18.	Farsighted	18._____	r.	tinea
19.	Ringworm	19._____	s.	toxic
20.	Syphilis	20._____	t.	ulcus

MEDICAL TERMS WHICH SOUND ALIKE

. The medical terms in each of the following pairs of words sound similar and are sometimes confused. Write the definition of each term in the space provided.

1. perineum   _____

   peritoneum   _____

2. mucus   _____

   mucous   _____

3. callus   _____

   callous   _____

4. ileum   _____

   ilium   _____

5. ureter   _____
   urethra   _____

6. aural

    oral

    _____

    _____

7. aphagia

    aphasia

    _____

    _____

8. cirrhosis

    scirrhous

    _____

    _____

9. abduction

    adduction

    _____

    _____

10. afferent

    efferent

    _____

    _____

11. pyogenic

    pyrogenic

    _____

    _____

12. stoma

    stroma

    _____

    _____

MEDICAL TERMS WHICH ARE OPPOSITES OR UNLIKES

A. For each medical term in the left hand column below, select the word that has an opposite or a distinctly different meaning from the column on the right and write the word in the answer column.

MEDICAL TERM	ANSWER	OPPOSITE OR UNLIKE WORD
1. Acute	1._____	a. acid
2. Alkali	2._____	b. acquired
3. Atrophy	3._____	c. alopecia
4. Autonomic	4._____	d. binary fission
5. Benign	5._____	e. chronic
6. Caudal	6._____	f. cranial
7. Congenital	7._____	g. epidemic
8. Distal	8._____	h. growth

9.	Dorsal	9._____	i.	malignant
10.	Endemic	10._____	j.	manifest
11.	Exacerbate	11._____	k.	mitigate
12.	Hirsute	12._____	l.	origin
13.	Immunity	13._____	m.	patent
14.	Insertion	14._____	n.	proximal
15.	Latent	15._____	o.	psychic
16.	Mitosis	16._____	p.	stroma
17.	Occluded	17._____	q.	supine
18.	Parenchyma	18._____	r.	susceptibility
19.	Prone	19._____	s.	ventral
20.	Somatic	20._____	t.	voluntary

B. In the space after each of the following medical terms, write the term that sounds partly the same but has opposite or distinctly different meaning (Example: inferior - superior).

MEDICAL TERM	OPPOSITE OR DISTINCTLY DIFFERENT TERM	MEDICAL TERM	OPPOSITE OR DISTINCTLY DIFFERENT TERM
1. afferent	_____	9. flexor	_____
2. androgen	_____	10. hypertension	_____
3. ante-partum	_____	11. inspiration	_____
4. anterior	_____	12. in vitro	_____
5. bradycardia	_____	13. multipara	_____
6. catabolism	_____	14. pronation	_____
7. endogenous	_____	15. septic	_____
8. eversion	_____	16. solute	_____

MEDICAL TERMS—SPELLING

A. Each of the following medical terms is spelled two ways: correctly and incorrectly. Write the correct spelling in the space provided.

MEDICAL TERM		CORRECT SPELLING
1. abscess	abcess	_____
2. aneurysm	anuerysm	_____

3.	antegen	antigen
4.	anteacid	antacid
5.	axillia	axilla
6.	barrium	barium
7.	bilirubin	billiruben
8.	bursitis	brusitis
9.	cateract	cataract
10.	cecum	ceccum
11.	cirhosis	cirrhosis
12.	clavical	clavicle
13.	colligen	collagen
14.	condile	condyle
15.	coxa	cocsa
16.	coxycs	coccyx
17.	debridment	debridement
18.	dermatitis	dermetitis
19.	diuretic	dieuretic
20.	dyspnea	dispnea

B. One spelling of the following medical terms is correct and the other incorrect. Write the correct spelling in the space provided.

	MEDICAL TERM	CORRECT SPELLING		MEDICAL TERM	CORRECT SPELLING
1.	eczema		6.	femur	
	excema			femour	
2.	endocrine		7.	furuncle	
	endocrin			feruncle	
3.	epiglottis		8.	hemaglobin	
	epiglotis			hemoglobin	
4.	epinephrine		9.	hirsuit	
	epinepherin			hirsute	
5.	erythemia		10.	homeostatis	
	erythema			homostasis	

226

11.	hydrocele		16.	malignent	
	hydroceel	_____		malignant	_____
12.	impetigo		17.	maxillia	
	impetego	_____		maxilla	_____
13.	inguinal		18.	metastasis	
	inguinul	_____		metastisis	_____
14.	ketone		19.	migrane	
	keytone	_____		migraine	_____
15.	labrynth		20.	murmur	
	labyrinth	_____		murmour	_____

C. One spelling of the following medical terms is correct and the other incorrect. Write the correct spelling in the space provided.

	MEDICAL TERM	CORRECT SPELLING		MEDICAL TERM	CORRECT SPELLING
1.	ophthalamic		11.	prurulent	
	ophthalmic	_____		purulent	_____
2.	orifice		12.	rale	
	orofice	_____		rahl	_____
3.	palour		13.	safranine	
	pallor	_____		saffronine	_____
4.	paroxsism		14.	scatoma	
	paroxysm	_____		scotoma	_____
5.	pertussis		15.	sinovitis	
	pertusis	_____		synovitis	_____
6.	plantor		16.	stuper	
	plantar	_____		stupor	_____
7.	polyp		17.	tempel	
	pollyp	_____		temple	_____
8.	postpartum		18.	tetenus	
	postpartem	_____		tetanus	_____
9.	protein		19.	varicose	
	protien	_____		varicous	_____
10.	proxamal		20.	venous	
	proximal	_____		venus	_____

MEDICAL TERMS FOR TYPES OF BODY STRUCTURE OR TISSUE

A. Match each of the following definitions of types of body structure or tissue
    with the correct term. Write the correct term in the answer column.

	DEFINITION	ANSWER		TERM
1.	A partition	1._____	a.	condyle
2.	An opening into the body	2._____	b.	cortex
3.	A pit or depression	3._____	c.	fascia
4.	Covering for synovial joints	4._____	d.	fossa
5.	Groove or furrow	5._____	e.	fundus
6.	Seam at junction of symmetrical parts	6._____	f.	hyaline
7.	Wrinkle, fold, or ridge	7._____	g.	lumen
8.	Ring of muscles controlling body opening	8._____	h.	meatus
9.	Outer layer of an organ	9._____	i.	plexus
10.	Fibrous sheath	10._____	j.	ramus
11.	Part farthest away from opening of an organ	11._____	k.	raphe
12.	Rounded eminence on end of bone	12._____	l.	ruga
13.	Branch from a larger part	13._____	m.	septum
14.	Network of nerves or vessels	14._____	n.	sphincter
15.	Space inside a tube or blood vessel	15._____	o.	sulcus

MEDICAL TERMS FOR TYPES OF BODY DISORDERS

A. Match the following definitions of body disorders with the proper medical term i
    the right-hand column. Write the term in the answer column.

	DEFINITION	ANSWER		MEDICAL TERM
1.	Excessive intercellular fluid	1._____	a.	abscess
2.	Escape of fluid into cavity or tissue	2._____	b.	adhesion
3.	Abnormal passage between organs or to exterior of body	3._____	c.	atrophy

4. Abnormal increase in size of an organ due to enlarged cells

4._____

d. cirrhosis

5. Death of tissue

5._____

e. edema

6. Slight paralysis

6._____

f. effusion

7. Alteration of form or function of tissue due to disease or injury

7._____

g. embolism

8. Local accumulation of pus

8._____

h. fistula

9. Formation of blood clot within the blood vessels

9._____

i. hernia

10. Occlusion of blood vessel by blood clot or foreign material

10._____

j. hypertrophy

11. Reduced local blood supply

11._____

k. hypoplasia

12. Coagulation of dead tissue due to inadequate blood supply

12._____

l. infarct

13. Abnormal connective tissue

13._____

m. ischemia

14. A spasm

14._____

n. lesion

15. Hardening of tissue

15._____

o. necrosis

16. Abnormal protrusion through containing wall

16._____

p. paresis

17. Drooping position of part

17._____

q. paroxysm

18. Reduction in size of organ or part

18._____

r. ptosis

19. Underdevelopment of organ or part

19._____

s. sclerosis

20. Inflammation of interstitial tissue

20._____

t. thrombosis

MEDICAL TERMS FOR SURGICAL PROCEDURES

A. Match each of the following definitions of surgical procedures by selecting the correct medical term from the right-hand column. Write the term in the answer column.

DEFINITION	ANSWER	TERM
1. Removal of living tissue for diagnostic study	1._____	a. anastomosis
2. Removing dead tissue and foreign material from wound	2._____	b. biopsy
3. Remove an entire organ	3._____	c. cautery
4. Scrape off tissue	4._____	d. cesarean sectio
5. Tying off a blood vessel	5._____	e. conization
6. Coagulation of tissue with heat or chemical	6._____	f. curettage
7. Tapping a cavity to draw off fluid	7._____	g. debridement
8. Creating an unnatural opening between two vessels or organs	8._____	h. enucleate
9. Cutting out a cone-shaped piece of tissue	9._____	i. excision
10. Abdominal incision to remove fetus	10._____	j. fulguration
11. General term for cutting out a part or tissue	11._____	k. herniorrhaphy
12. Cutting into the body	12._____	l. incision
13. Destruction of tissue with electric sparks	13._____	m. ligation
14. Suturing for repair of hernia	14._____	n. lithotomy
15. Incision to remove a stone from a duct or organ	15._____	o. paracentesis